"I applaud Joni's delightful and exhaustive (pun intended) approach to overcoming this ever increasing problem of insomnia in today's hectic society."

—**PAUL SCHEINBERG, MD, FCCP**

Dr. Paul Scheinberg, currently serving as Chief Medical Officer of Emory Saint Joseph's Hospital of Atlanta, is the Founding Partner of Atlanta Pulmonary Group, a Private Practice of physicians Board Certified in Pulmonary, Critical Care, and/or Sleep Medicine. He has made appearances on CNN, NBC and other outlets on a variety of topics.

NURSE, NURSE, I'M WORSE!

CAN YOU HELP ME SLEEP?

Joni Bellew, RN

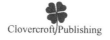
Clovercroft Publishing

Published by Clovercroft Publishing, Franklin, Tennessee.

Published in association with Larry Carpenter of Christian Book Services, LLC. www.christianbookservices.com

Scripture taken from the NEW AMERICAN STANDARD BIBLE®, Copyright © 1960,1962,1963,1968,1971,1972,1973,1975,1977,1995 by The Lockman Foundation. Used by permission.

Edited by Lapiz Digital Services

Cover Illustration by Laura Nuse

Cover and Interior Layout Design by Suzanne Lawing

Printed in the United States of America

978-1-945507-17-5

Table of Contents

A song for sleep

—Exercises: physical, mental, and breathing activities to induce sleep
—Emotional fitness for improving sleep quality
—Exercising joy as the fruit of being rested and energized
—Educating others to live energized and externally focused as a servant

PREFACE

While attending the Capstone College of Nursing, I frequently came home on the weekends to spend time with my family. Barely taking time to park my Roll Tide—crimson and white—Plymouth Horizon, I opened the sliding glass doors and entered the scene announcing, "I'm home!" Like a wounded soldier, I could hear my dad echo from some random corner of the house, *"Nurse, Nurse, I'm Worse!"*

Of course, he was perfectly fine. This was just his mischievously endearing way of saying, *"Welcome home, Daddy's girl—soon to be nurse!"*

It was our fun little ritual.

Although I much preferred the study of journalism, my dad controlled the purse strings. He would tell me, in reference to journalism and the liberal news media, *"That industry will eat you alive."* Therefore, my second choice—plan B—for a college major, was teaching. I wanted to be an English or History teacher. As a result, Dad would frequently open the *Want Ads* and point to one nursing job after the next, commenting disparagingly, "Teachers are a dime a dozen."

With the king's money, comes the king—so, like a lamb being led to the slaughter, I went for a nursing degree—enduring every minute of the pursuit. To this day, my dad's ultimate goal of keeping me steadily and gainfully employed is being fulfilled. Ironically, I've actually enjoyed my nursing career, in part, because I didn't choose the traditional nursing model.

Years later, after earning my Bachelor of Science in Nursing (BSN) and becoming a Registered Nurse (RN), I was diagnosed with Grave's disease. My arduous journey back to wholeness took a few detours, but I overcame this autoimmune disorder through nutrition and life-style changes. Once I rejected the conventional treatment plan of allopathic medicine, and chose to, as Hippocrates famously admonished—*let food be my medicine, and medicine be my food*—I reached my destination of total wellness.

The day I called my dad to tell him my labs were all normal, he was thrilled, and we were both truly grateful. My dad lovingly challenged, "God will require something of you. He will want you to share the wisdom you've gained so others can be healed." How interesting of my dad to make such a declaration!

The truth is, while I was sick, I did not have the faith to ask for healing, but I did possess enough faith to ask for the wisdom necessary to forge my own path to wellness. Along the way, I eventually learned that healing and wisdom are most often synonymous.

This book is the culmination of all I have learned in my personal walk with God on my journey from sickness to health. Based on my own experience, sweet, restorative sleep is one of the fruits of a life that's well-orchestrated and well-lived. If you are living a balanced, optimal life-style, sleep will come easily and be a faithful friend. Thus, the title of the book, *Nurse, Nurse, I'm Worse! Can You Help Me Sleep?*

My mom, being well-read, imparted to me her love for books—as well as her ferocious appetite for stories from gifted authors. At any given moment of the day, she can be found in her favorite chair reading her latest find. For years she has encouraged me to write and to this day she tells me, "You should have been a journalist." Perhaps life-style coaching will be the springboard of my writing career as a literary missionary—and recapture what might have been.

To write a book like this requires the wisdom of God and the help of numerous talented people. I would like to thank Jack Watts for mentoring me throughout the entire process, including the long hours of editing. He also introduced me to an amazingly gifted team of people, Anne Alexander, Dwayne Bassett, Patty Fitts, Colin Hawk, and Larry A. Carpenter, along with Suzanne Lawing. I also want to thank my personal friend, Laura Nuse. Thank you to each one of you for your part in helping me write and create this book.

I'm on a mission—a mission to put *you* to sleep. One way or the other, this book is sure to do it. Wink!

INTRODUCTION

Holiday is one of my all-time favorite movies. It's a whimsical tale, centered around two women who need to make serious changes in their lives. Although they live on opposite sides of the Atlantic Ocean, they decide to swap houses during the holiday season, which changes their lives forever and for the better.

While putting this book together, it occurred to me that Amanda's character (played by Cameron Diaz) and her storyline as an insomniac, who has lost the ability to cry, embodies everything I want to illustrate in this book.

You may ask yourself, "Do I need to make a course correction like Amanda?" Perhaps you do. You too, might be one of the millions of overstimulated people, living on too much sugar and caffeine—just to function—after cheating yourself of needed sleep from the previous night.

Seemingly, there is a lack of understanding—especially with millennials—in knowing the importance of powering down at night. People of all ages are experiencing sleep loss, and in some cases, severe sleep deprivation. However, the toll this problem is taking on our children—as well as our teens—is especially alarming. Once you learn how important sleep is, and you consider the immediate—as well as the long-term consequences of skimping on sleep—you'll be motivated to stop at nothing to get your needed Zzz's.

Although, Amanda's sleep issues vanish once her dream man shows up—this typical "reel" Hollywood answer to every woman's problems is most likely not the "real" answer to your sleep issues. It certainly was not the answer to my own battle with sleep loss. In fact, meeting the love of your life can actually bring unique sleeping challenges that may complicate your life—and in some cases, wreak full-blown havoc on your sleep.

New relationships often require an adjustment phase, to ward off potential sleep disruptions. Making a concerted effort to synchronize both you and your partner's sleep patterns might be difficult at first, but the rewards of sharing your life with a loving companion are well worth the effort.

Whether insomnia visits you on rare occasions—or it rudely came to stay without an invitation—there is much to learn concerning restorative sleep.

I'm going to challenge you to remodel your life—much like Amanda remodeled her life. The process begins with the simple question, "What's keeping you up at night?" When Amanda pondered this very question, it resulted in a big exchange of swapping houses. Let's walk this back and revisit Amanda at the onset of her journey in conquering debilitating insomnia. It looks like she's really losing it. Can't you hear her pleading, *"Nurse, Nurse, I'm Worse! Can you help me sleep?"*

To that urgent cry, I say, "Yes, Amanda, I thought you would never ask. I can help you!"

And I can help you too, dear reader.

Nick Saban, the head Football Coach at the University of Alabama, as well as, five-time and counting, National Championship winner, teaches his team the power of "the process." My approach to coaching clients to better sleep utilizes a similar concept, "the *Nursing Process*," which I learned while earning my BSN from The University of Alabama, Capstone College of Nursing. This process—yielding the same winning results as the Alabama Crimson Tide—involves APIE:

- **A**ssessing the problem
- **P**lanning through a written care plan
- **I**mplementing the care plan
- **E**valuating outcomes

Additionally, my unique approach to restorative sleep is based on my comprehensive coaching model, using the N.U.R.S.E. acronym. As I promote optimal living, I believe *sleep* is the ultimate barometer for measuring desired outcomes from these five distinct categories. Each of the following categories, if properly managed, will yield restorative sleep:

- Nutrition
- Uncluttering
- Remodeling
- Spirituality
- Exercise

Think of me as your very own N.U.R.S.E. coach. With my nursing bag full of paraphernalia, I want to inspire you to re-order your out-of-balance life—so, you can live optimally and sleep like a baby.

There is no way around the fact that I am truly a southern belle at the core of my being—straight from the Heart of Dixie, born and bred in the Bible Belt. Perhaps I'm a dying breed, but I'm a good 'ole *Girl Reered in the South (G.R.I.T.S)*. Women of the South are gentile and soft but we have grit—thus, the term steel magnolias. We love our Bibles, beau's and our babies like fierce mama bears. When I tell you this southern culture possesses some tried and true remedies for insomnia, you can believe me. The Bible verses, old hymns, gospel music, and Scripture lullabies of the Deep South are some of the best remedies you'll find for quietening your soul and partaking of restful sleep.

My dear granny imparted her faith to me, and I wouldn't trade that for anything in this world. If you were at her house, she would tell you, just as she used to tell me, "Sleep in peace, knowing you have nothing to fear." As a result of my rich heritage, I learned how to tackle the insomnia problem full on.

Toss the Hollywood "reel" answers—such as finding your soulmate—as a cure-all for problems that are robbing you of precious sleep. Romantic love may have helped our fictitious Hollywood character, Amanda, but true insomnia, as my granny knew, is often a spiritual matter. The good news, however, is—the One who created you, and desires a "real" relationship with you, has the answer to the problem of insomnia.

One of the names for God in the Scriptures is Jehovah Rohi—your heavenly Shepherd. Did you ever stop to think that while you sleep, He works the night shift on your behalf? Jehovah Rohi is shepherding your life, so you don't have to do anything but sleep. Instead of counting sheep to help you fall asleep, count your blessings and your Zzz's, allowing our Lord to count you among the sheep of His flock.

The Scriptures reveal He even counts the number of hairs on your head. How attentive and loving He is towards you. Choosing to maintain the mindset that you are His little lamb in the heavenly sheepfold—benefits you endlessly—starting with a well-rested life.

If you skip any section of this book, you may just miss the one truth that holds the key to curing your insomnia. It may seem that drinking too much coffee is the reason you can't sleep, but what is causing you to drink so much coffee? After it is all said and done, don't be surprised if the root of your insomnia turns out to be something other than the obvious.

To see if this holds true for you, let's get started with assessing what's really keeping you up at night.

P.S. Look for the *Sleep Q-Tips* icon:

Nurses have a host of paraphernalia we use to care for our patients—blood pressure cuffs, thermometers, stethoscopes, and bandaids, just to name a few. I, for one, love the Q-tip for swabbing ears and wound care, as well as, for grooming and bathing babies. That's why I have a magic Q-tip that is ready to swab away your insomnia—much like a fairy godmother waves her wand and makes everything better.

At the end of each chapter, I will list tips to help you improve your quality of sleep under the heading "Sleep Q-Tips" (Q for quality). So look for the Q-Tip icon for a brief summary and quick reference at the close of each section. My magic Q-Tip helps to eliminate insomnia, allowing you to count your blessings and your Zzz's, instead of those annoying *baaaad* sheep at night.

PART I

Restorative Sleep

AMANDA: OUR INSOMNIAC AND HER CHALLENGES

Sleep is a precious, rare commodity these days. More and more, people of all ages are sleep deprived, and it's taking a huge toll on our society. Despite a rapidly growing sleep industry—spanning the gamut from pharmaceuticals to a wide array of luxurious bedding, we still toss and turn throughout the night. Even with an assortment of innovative mattresses that are covered with the finest linens money can buy and the most comfy sleepwear manufactured to date—sleep seems to escape our grasp.

Take Amanda, for example, in a scene from *Holiday*. Even though her bedroom is fit for a royal princess, equipped with soft lighting, remote-controlled window shades that totally darken the room—and an interior design that would allow anyone to snooze in peace for days—Amanda is powerless to fall asleep.

She lives in a freestanding dream house on a quiet street in Los Angeles—not a noisy high-rise in a big city that never sleeps. Whatever is sabotaging her efforts to sleep each night is not environmental. So, it remains to be seen what is actually keeping her up at night. Is she suffering from an unknown endogenous issue? Let's see how this unfolds for Amanda.

Notwithstanding her best efforts, Amanda's mind torments her all night with jingles playing over and over in her head—a frustrating work hazard from creating advertising ads all day. Sleepless nights, like those Amanda experiences, have potential long-term consequences that require immediate attention.

Here's where I come in . . .

Perhaps just like Amanda you're saying, "Nurse, Nurse, I'm Worse!" You may be wearily inquiring, "Can you help me sleep?"

I hear this all the time from a myriad of individuals suffering from a lack of sleep. And the answer is a resounding, "Yes! I can help you!"

But be warned. Because I care about you, I'm going to be the Sleep Police! You need way more sleep than you realize, and my role is to help you get that needed sleep. When it comes to teaching you the importance of sleep satiation—a state of feeling completely and fully rested with perfect recall of the previous night's dream(s)—my approach is militant. Being intentional about enjoying a full night's sleep is the single most important action you can take towards slowing down the aging process, and it will also help you prevent a host of age-related maladies, such as, Alzheimer's disease and dementia.

When you sleep soundly throughout the night, your body produces somatotropin, the growth hormone, which works to repair damage from the normal wear and tear of the day. Just think of it, this wonderful thing you do, called sleep, is completely free. It doesn't cost you a dime, but the benefits are endless.

I am not ashamed to tell you that I need nine hours of sleep, as well as an occasional nap, to experience sleep satiation. It's a way of life for me. My skin tells on me and so will yours—if you routinely cheat yourself of healthy sleep. Without restorative sleep, the vessels under your eyes dilate, causing blood to pool in this delicate area. Additionally this leads to unattractive puffiness, known as "bags under your eyes." In the absence of sleep, you lose moisture in your face, which causes your skin to sag due to dehydration. Also, due to hormonal imbalances, skin breakouts often occur.

Because I care about you, I am going to be a zealot when it comes to coaching you to a fantastic "sleep" life. I want you to look fresh, feel rested, and sport a fit physique, while possessing clarity of mind and a vibrant, patient personality. No one wants to be around a fat, foggy, sleep-deprived curmudgeon, do you?

Researchers tell us the more sleep you forego, the harder it is for adults to lose belly fat. Dr. Daniel Amen, in his Alzheimer's and dementia research, concludes that the bigger the belly, the smaller the brain—referring to this phenomenon as the "dinosaur syndrome."

The good news, according to Dr. Amen, is once his plan is followed and changes occur, such as a considerable reduction in abdominal fat, erosive patches of brain tissue, attributed to dementia and Alzheimer's—in almost all cases—can be notably reversed (www.brainwarriorswaycourse.com).

Without adequate sleep, as you age, it is difficult to lose stubborn belly fat. Therefore, with consistent, restful sleep, it is believed, your chances of developing dementia and Alzheimer's are significantly reduced and successful minimization of belly fat is more readily achieved.

Because Alzheimer's begins decades before there are any outward signs and symptoms, you may think you are getting away with hours of foregone sleep, but the toll does not always show up immediately. Recall Amanda—even though she's in her late twenties or early thirties—by missing out on sound, restorative sleep, you too, could be setting yourself up for Alzheimer's. More often than not, serious long-term, residual sleep deprivation takes years to develop. In addition to Alzheimer's, chronic sleep loss puts you at risk for a host of other potential maladies:

- Heart attack
- Heart disease
- Heart failure
- Irregular heartbeat
- High blood pressure
- Stroke
- Diabetes

Up to 90% of people with insomnia have additional health issues (www.webmd.com/sleep-disorders/excessive-sleepiness-10/10-results-sleep-loss).

There will always be a new study, here or there, claiming you don't need as much sleep as once thought, but the research, so far, that has stood the test of time, lines up with the obvious. God gave you 24 hours each day, with a portion of the day ending at sunset for sleep, and a sunrise for awaking—at, or near dawn. Your circadian rhythm is designed to work in sync with this cycle.

In fact, a recent study released in June of 2016 reveals this very phenomenon. According to the researchers at Northwestern University Chicago, people that travel between time zones or work rotating shifts are at a higher risk for heart attacks. This study stresses the importance of a regular, routine sleep schedule if you want to protect your heart (www.dailymail.co.uk/health/article-3627647/Going-bed-time-night-reduces-risk-heart-disease.html).

Related to protecting your heart, recall Amanda's sleep problems. Ironically, they are in part, a matter of the heart, potentially affecting her in a physical capacity. Ultimately, if left unchecked, her sleep deprivation could result in all sorts of maladies that Amanda does not want to experience—nor do you. Let's take a look at some additional unintended consequences of chronic sleep loss.

A CONTINUED REVIEW OF INSOMNIA: ADDITIONAL CAUSES AND RESULTING MALADIES

It is important for you to get on with the business of sleep—to potentially reverse any existing damage and ward off future harm—as a result of chronic sleep loss. Ask yourself the following questions:

"Have I been getting enough sleep for the past decade(s)?"

"How much sleep do I need to feel completely rested?"

"Have I been skimping on sleep lately, possibly risking, at the very least, the development of a bad habit?"

Or worse yet, "Am I already living a sleep-deprived lifestyle?"

Exhaustion begets exhaustion, so it's important to get in the sleep zone and stay there. Unfortunately, the people that need sleep the most are the ones who can't sleep. It's just like your bank account. Once you overdraw from your sleep account, you continue to make choices that cause you to run up a deficit—putting your account in the red for Zzz's. Loading up on caffeine and other stimulants—in a desperate attempt to stay falsely energized throughout the day—results in adrenal exhaustion. Thus, the downward spiral begins.

ADRENAL EXHAUSTION DUE TO STIMULANTS AND ELECTRONICS

Adrenal exhaustion is, in part, a byproduct of all the coffee bars sprinkled along every street corner. You are part of a culture that drinks more coffee now than ever before. And what is worse, these coffee drinks are loaded with cream and sugar—from the simplest cup of coffee to a whole spectrum of designer coffees, such as lattes and cappuccinos. Caffeinated specialty drinks are dehydrating and fattening, as well as stimulating. They power you up, when you are burning it at both ends. Then, when you need to power down and fall asleep, you simply can't unwind. You're wired from toxic caffeine overload.

Why is sleep deprivation at an all-time high? The answer lies beyond the obvious reasons already mentioned. It's a fact that artificial light, glowing throughout the bedroom from the television, computers, and other hand-held devices, actually destroys your melatonin. This naturally occurring hormone in the body, which declines significantly after age 30, is designed to trigger sleep. Even after you decide to turn the lights off and get some sleep, if you leave the TV flickering in the background, you'll hamper the brain's ability to signal the release of sleep hormones—especially melatonin.

The good news is everyday new products are announced to help diminish the destructive blue lighting from electronics that destroys melatonin, such as the GE Align PM Light Bulb. Blue light detected by a unique group of cells in the eye impacts our melatonin levels. This low-blue comfort light, intended for evening use before bedtime, helps maintain sleep rhythms by varying the blue content of light, while promoting the body's natural sleep cycle.

The best product I've found for anyone who feels they must be on the computer late at night is the Uvex Skyper Blue Light Blocking Computer Glasses with spectrum control technology (SCT)–Orange Lens (S1933X). These night time goggles are a godsend, if you are married to a computer late at night. They sell for under $10.00. The Orange Lens features SCT to absorb 98% or more of the blue light emitted from laptops, computers, iPads, etc. The result is an additional screen contrast with sharpened details, which improves focus, reduces eye fatigue, and helps inhibit vision problems, such as cataracts and age-related macular degeneration.

There will continue to be improved technology available to you for late night use of hand held devices, but even so, it is better to remember the natural sleep pattern and stick with the circadian rhythm God gave us. Even if the blue light issue is remedied and melatonin levels are not diminished, you still need to put all the gadgets down and sleep.

In the days before electricity, people went to bed when the sun set and got up with the chickens at dawn. Their bodies were in tune with natural sunlight, so they got plenty of sleep after a hard day of physical labor. Although they fell into bed tired, it was a "good" tired. You now have a new kind of exhaustion, resulting from too much stress and a sedentary life-style.

Perhaps your adrenals are blown as a result of sipping on stimulating, sweet coffee drinks throughout the day, while staring at artificial light from a host of electronic devices. Society expects this so you can push yourself beyond your limit mentally—to perform for hours on end, while you sacrifice precious sleep.

If you suspect you have adrenal exhaustion, go to the following website and take the adrenal test: https://www.adrenalfatigue.org/take-the-adrenal-fatigue-quiz. If it reads, "Oops this page cannot be found," look for the tab at the top that's labeled: Take the Adrenal Fatigue Quiz. You can calculate your score and determine to what degree you are experiencing adrenal fatigue.

Another contributing factor to today's sleep deprivation is that previous generations rarely ate sweets. When they did have something sweet, it was in a more natural form, such as seasonal fruit, maple syrup, or honey—and a well-deserved treat. Today, sugar is part of every meal, plus snacks throughout the day. Unlike this generation, your ancestors, as recently as your grandparents, ate smart and were active all day. So, by sundown, their bodies were ready to receive restful, restorative sleep. They didn't fight sleep—they welcomed it.

CHILDREN AND SLEEP

Children are naturally more able to sleep, due to ample levels of melatonin, but they too are being compromised by all of the technology. More and more children operate with a sleep deficit, affecting their overall growth and development. Especially at risk is their immune system.

When I was in nursing school, we were taught the first six years of a child's life are critical, as they are building their foundation for a healthy immune system. Going with the assumption that this teaching still stands today, I believe the first five to six years of a child's life are fundamental—in their overall development and consequentially, their ability to fight future diseases throughout their lives.

Children need lots of sound sleep in order to build the strongest foundation possible. This ensures they have the necessary building blocks for a robust immune system to support them for years to come, carrying them into a bright healthy future. Kathi Kemper, MD, Director of the Center for Holistic Pediatric Education and Research at Children's Hospital in

Boston, is an avid speaker and writer, promoting healthy habits for our children. She also believes our children need more sleep.

How would you like to wake up fully rested, eager to get down the hall and wake up the kids—only to find they are already busy getting dressed for the day? Does this sound like a fairy-tale? The norm doesn't have to be fighting every day of the week, just to get your children, especially teens, out the door and off to school. If they were afforded a little more time to recoup from staying up too late, in their overstimulated world, they might be more cooperative in the morning.

The National Sleep Foundation's website, www.sleepfoundation.org, has suggested schools should start at least 45 minutes later every day. One school moved the start time from 7:30 to 8:15 a.m. (In my opinion, 7:30 is way too early.) Other schools started a full hour later. Of the schools that signed up for the change, the following has occurred:

- More alert and engaged students
- Grades trending upward
- Improved moods/attitudes
- Less drop-outs
- A decrease in call outs
- Reports of less depression among students
- Fewer discipline problems
- Better health, less illness
- Happier students, teachers, and parents

Our youth are developing very unnatural sleep patterns by consistently going to bed too late. Computers and Internet games—so prevalent in today's electronic culture—allow their young minds to do mental gymnastics way into the night. This puts their growing, revved up brains into overload. It was intended, from the beginning of time, that you start winding down, mentally and physically, around sunset. It is important to understand that just because "lights out" is announced, the mind can't automatically switch gears and instantly shut down. Children need the proper preparation for going to bed earlier, and they need to sleep later in the morning for their overall growth and development.

A teacher at Wilson Elementary in Kenosha, Wisconsin, has raised the rhetoric and the national conversation for the hot topic of how much sleep a child needs. She posted a sleep chart on Facebook resulting in over 400,000 hits and the number of hits continues to grow. Experts, such as Jodi Mindell, a psychology professor and sleep expert at St. Joseph's University, endorsed the chart. Mindell states the chart is congruent with the "10 under 10" rule. Kids under 10 years of age need at least 10 hours of sleep. According to Mindell, "Multiple studies show that children who go to bed before 9 get much more

At what time should your child go to bed?

Age	Wake-up time						
---	6:00 AM	6:15 AM	6:30 AM	6:45 AM	7:00 AM	7:15 AM	7:30 AM
	Sleeping time						
5	6:45 PM	7:00 PM	7:15 PM	7:30 PM	7:30 PM	8:00 PM	8:15 PM
6	7:00 PM	7:15 PM	7:30 PM	7:30 PM	8:00 PM	8:15 PM	8:30 PM
7	7:15 PM	7:15 PM	7:30 PM	8:00 PM	8:15 PM	8:30 PM	8:45 PM
8	19:30	7:30 PM	8:00 PM	8:15 PM	8:30 PM	8:45 PM	9:00 PM
9	7:30 PM	8:00 PM	8:15 PM	8:30 PM	8:45 PM	9:00 PM	9:15 PM
10	8:00 PM	8:15 PM	8:30 PM	8:45 PM	9:00 PM	9:15 PM	9:30 PM
11	8:15 PM	8:30 PM	8:45 PM	9:00 PM	9:15 PM	9:30 PM	9:45 PM
12	8:15 PM	8:30 PM	8:45 PM	9:00 PM	9:15 PM	9:30 PM	9:45 PM

sleep than those who go to bed later than 9."

Parents, you need to lead by example. Monitor your children, and shut down all electronic gadgets, at least an hour before bed, preferably several hours in advance of retiring. We all need to allow our bodies to transition from the fast pace of the day into a quiet, more settled, nightly ritual, conducive to sleep. When you skimp on sleep, the family suffers, and the household becomes irritable and short tempered. This is not the best atmosphere for rearing healthy children, nor is it a recipe for creating a happy home. No one wants to be around grumpy people with short fuses because they don't get enough Zzz's. When you power down and prepare for sleep, everyone wins. But this dynamic does not happen by osmosis. You have to be intentional and work to make it happen. It is worth it. I promise.

Common sense would tell you, anyone who gets too little or too much sleep is probably not going to function as well as someone who gets the recommended amount of sleep. The amount varies for individuals, depending on age. With too little sleep, your inhibitions are down, so naturally you're not as able to withstand temptation. With too much sleep, you may need to consider depression as a potential root cause. A tired person is more weak-willed. But add to that, the immortal thinking of teenagers, and the idea that they are, in their minds, invincible. There's definitely cause for added concern.

It is no surprise that teens, foregoing the right amount of sleep, are more prone to risk-taking and dangerous behaviors—such as driving drunk and succumbing to peer pressure. However, the CDC released a study in early 2016 that confirms this very finding: *CDC—Teens with Sleep Issues More Often Take Dangerous Risks*, by Mike Stobbe, Associated Press.

MILLENNIALS AND SLEEP

Arianna Huffington is so concerned about the rampant

sleep deprivation occurring across the country on college campuses that she launched a Sleep Revolution tour. She's teaching young sleep-deprived souls that they need to disconnect—at least for eight full hours—and actually sleep. The millennials are afraid they will miss a text or tweet, or the latest tidbit of gossip on Facebook, so they are simply sleep starved. They don't know how to disconnect. They can be exhausted but if they get on a device late at night, they'll be up until the wee hours of the morning. It was Arianna that introduced me to the current term, FOMO—Fear Of Missing Out.

Speaking of fear, I just met a girl at the Apple store who suffers from oneirophobia—fear of dreams. Also, she claims to suffer from somniphobia, hypnophobia, and cliniphobia—all names for fear of sleep. She does not know why this irrational and excessive fear developed during her college years. Nothing significant comes to her mind as to what might have been a trigger. A decade later, she drinks Slippery Elm, tea from a tree bark, to help her sleep—and she swears by it. She also wears a sleep hood with speakers for listening to sleep apps that help induce sleep.

One thing we both agreed on—she has a very creative mind that she constantly keeps in a revved up mode. Today's culture and her profession do not help her sleep.

In addition to this overstimulated IT culture, let's circle back to all the additives, preservatives, and stimulants—such as sugar in your food and beverages. Cutting back on these items, or eliminating them all together, is a strong step in the right direction. Unless your body is prepared for sleep through proper nutrition, and you've created a quiet environment, it will not be restful sleep—even if sleep actually comes.

BLOOD SUGAR AND SLEEP

Lynn Maarouf, RD (Registered Dietician), Education Director of the Stark Diabetes Center at the University of Texas

Medical Branch in Galveston, encourages her clients to eat properly throughout the day—so they can better control their glucose levels, yielding a better night's sleep. Maarouf says, "If you get your blood sugars under control, you can sleep great throughout the night and wake up feeling energized." She goes on to say that frequent urination during the night is often the body's attempt to rid itself of excessive glucose levels in the bloodstream.

According to Mark Mahowald, Director of the Minnesota Regional Sleep Disorders Center, in Hennepin County, there is a relationship between insulin resistance—a precursor to Diabetes—and sleep deprivation. Diabetes is a disease where the cells do not properly make or regulate insulin. When insulin is not properly managed, you suffer a loss of energy and probable damage—eventually to one, or all, of the following: the kidneys, eyes, nerves and heart (www.webmd.com/sleep-disorders/excessive-sleepiness-10/diabetes-lack-of-sleep).

The purpose of sleep is to give the body a chance to restore itself from the wear and tear of the day. If the body is always digesting food while you sleep, because you gorged yourself before hitting the pillow, restoration will not occur. It is recommended that you have your biggest meal, no later than 4 p.m. and perhaps refrain from eating after 7 p.m., to avoid gaining weight, especially adults aged 30 and older. This is related to a naturally occurring, slower metabolism that comes with age.

There are many steps you can take to retard the aging process, but the most important one, is getting plenty of restful sleep, also known as—beauty sleep. The skin, as previously alluded to, is very telling, when you've cheated your body of sound sleep. So, keep the body in a state of rest rather than in a state of digesting, during nighttime slumber, maximizing rejuvenation.

In order to get restful sleep, it is equally important to avoid going to sleep on an empty stomach, unless this is a declared fast for cleansing, and that is a special circumstance. A declared fast would be more than 12 hours and is usually no less than 24 hours.

The word "breakfast" is from two words "break" and "fast." You should take a break from eating for 10 to 12 hours every day, between approximately 7 p.m. until 5 a.m. to 7 a.m., for the purpose of yielding optimal sleep conditions. Some people require a bite of cheese or peanut butter with a cracker, or milk and cereal right before bed. Fats and simple carbohydrates, with a little protein, keep the blood sugar stable. But eat nothing more, to avoid potential weight gain and insomnia. These small snacks release serotonin and help promote sleep (more on this in the N section: Nutrition).

Since you are tightening up your nighttime habits, no more dessert before bed. When insomnia is turning your life upside down, you have to focus on every aspect of life—until that nasty, sleep-killing monster is conquered. Making a strict course correction with a schedule and consistent habits is a must. But don't be too alarmed; I am a realist. I'll eventually build some wiggle room into your evening ritual. But for now we are full on! Stay with me. You will love your life so much more when you are fully rested.

COOLING DOWN FOR SLEEP

So, let's check in. How many cups of coffee have you consumed today? See if you can stick to one cup in the morning, upon awakening (two at the most) and then no more caffeine the rest of the day. I'm serious. You need sleep, and I'm here to see that nothing compromises your nighttime slumber. At least I didn't ask you to give up caffeine completely.

Another recommendation is to avoid having a smoke and then immediately crashing into bed at the end of the day.

Nicotine may relax your nerves, but it is also a stimulant. Let your body temperature drop by taking a shower and then perhaps air dry to cool down. Keep the room cool, so you can get the rest you need. Sleep loves a cooler environment, and your body may respond to sleep even after a smoke if the room is cooler.

Seems like the latest rage is to eat Paleo. So, if you can eat like a cave man, then you can sleep like a cave man. Sleep in the nude. The cooler the core of the body, the quicker you drift off to sleep. Tests reveal room temps of 66° and slightly above help your insulin levels stabilize, keeping your fat metabolism in the good fat zone. Temperatures of 81° and above are not healthy for optimal sleep. Make sure you have a temperature-appropriate room—not too cool or too hot—but cooler is better. The article, "Let's Cool It in the Bedroom," appeared in the July 20, 2014, issue of The New York Times Magazine (http://well.blogs.nytimes.com/2014/07/17/lets-cool-it-in-the-bedroom/?_r=0).

WINE AND SLEEP

For all of you wine lovers, here is a news flash. Perhaps wine is not the nightcap it is thought to be. Researchers have found that, although wine can aid you in drifting off to sleep, it interferes with the second cycle of sleep. You end up compromising the wonderful aspect of sleep called "dreaming" or rapid eye movement (REM) sleep. Wine can help you fall asleep now and then, but having a routine nightcap can backfire, if you are one of many people that builds up a tolerance. Therefore, the effect of a nightly glass of wine for the sole purpose of seeking a sleep aid is questionable, at best.

If you find you are not sleeping soundly, ask yourself, "Do I need to slow down on my evening wine consumption to improve my overall quality of sleep?" More than two glasses of wine in the evening can definitely hamper sleep. Several studies have concluded that drinking too much wine, in general, causes you to awaken much earlier than you should—thereby sabotaging your overall ability to acquire an adequate amount of sleep.

Sip and savor your glass of wine to stretch out the experience. Try taking slower more deliberate sips. Spend more time enjoying one glass of wine before going for another pour (www.prevention.com/health/sleep-energy/wine-can-sabotage-sleep-quality).

BEING INTENTIONAL ABOUT GETTING ENOUGH SLEEP

Most people only dream of getting a full eight hours of sleep at night, but the truth is you really need nine hours, especially if you suffer from adrenal exhaustion. Two hours of sleep before midnight is better than four hours after midnight.

In Jordan Rubin's must read book, *The Maker's Diet*, he reveals that healing hormones work the hardest to repair your body between 9 p.m. and midnight. Anyone fighting a disease should take note of this and try to be asleep by 9 p.m.—with the ultimate goal of sleeping uninterrupted, at the very least, through the midnight hour—but preferably the entire night. More specifically, Jordan tells us that every minute you sleep before midnight is the equivalent of four minutes of sleep after midnight.

Avoid working up a second wind before bedtime. When you start to feel tired, go with it. Don't push yourself until you get a second wind. If you have a lull and you nod off at 9 p.m., but you push yourself to stay up until 11 p.m. or midnight, this is not a healthy lifestyle. A night, here or there, will not take a huge toll on you, but if this is your modus operandi, then immediate changes need to occur. Don't clean the kitchen, walk the dog, or watch another TV program. By teaching your body to go with a second wind, and recharge for another round of chores, you train your body to fight sleep. (DVR shows and watch them the next day. Leave the dishes or plan ahead for kitchen cleaning. Know and respectfully listen to what your body is signaling.)

Everyone loves to wake up to a clean kitchen, so if it's late and you can't sleep with a dirty kitchen in the next room, join the "clean as you go" club. With intentionality, you can walk the dog, clean the kitchen, help the kids with their homework, or any other work-related task, and still make it to bed at a decent hour. The healthiest people go to bed early and get started early. Benjamin Franklin said, "Early to bed, early to rise, makes a man healthy, wealthy and wise."

If you are thinking, "I know this sounds doable but un-realistic—with the holidays approaching, out-of-town com-pany or other special occasions—this is going to be extremely challenging." Just remember when it comes to health, whether it is eating right or getting enough sleep, you can apply the 80/20 principle. Live intentionally 80% of the time and with the other 20% give yourself some wiggle room. When you continually ignore your body's cry for sleep, and chronically push yourself to the limit, it sets you up for disease. So, try as much as possible, to stay on a regular schedule due to the many benefits of living a consistent life-style, but don't stress if you have times where you have to compromise.

REM (RAPID EYE MOVEMENT) SLEEP AND THE BRAIN-GUT CONNECTION

Jordan writes in great length about the second brain, called the "gut," which is part of the enteric nervous system. The gut, or intestines, mimics the brain in the central nervous system, in that each organ has memory. Both the brain and the gut produce feelings. The central nervous system is seen as the primary nervous system, but the enteric nervous system is just as important. Through the connection of the longest cranial nerve—the vagus nerve—you get the vital brain-gut connection. That's where the term, "gut feelings" or "trusting your gut" originated. There is also the well-known reference to "butterflies in your stomach." I allude to these examples, because it helps you recognize your gut is attached to wisdom and thinking, just as the brain is.

Jordan makes the case that sleep is one of the greatest gifts you can give your "gut," which in the end promotes digestion and overall health. Have you ever suffered from a sour stomach after a sleepless night? Now you know why. It is fascinating and important to note that the brain and the gut both have 90-minute cycles. REM sleep of the brain is about 90 minutes and allows for deeper sleep so you can dream. People with irritable bowel syndrome and other bowel problems, including nonulcer dyspepsia or "sour stomach," often report suffering from poor sleep, along with insufficient REM sleep.

According to Dr. Archibald Hart in his book, *Adrenaline and Stress*, there are two types of sleep, REM or dreaming sleep and non-REM or nondreaming sleep. He tells you that people who have manual jobs need more non-REM sleep. People with thinking, but sedentary jobs, such as accountants, need more REM or dreaming sleep, because this helps the mind sort, organize, and prevent information overload.

Dream sleep or REM sleep is a much deeper sleep, whereby the body visibly reacts during this stage of sleep. You breathe more slowly and demonstrate REM, with your eyelids twitching and fluttering. Your fingers tend to grow cold while your toes become warmer. Your blood pressure falls rapidly, especially during the first three hours of sleep. Without ever knowing it, you can change positions during your sleep, from 20 to 60 times.

Every 90 minutes or so, you should slip into REM sleep from non-REM sleep. If you find that you are awake and need to go to the rest room, you could still be in a state of semiconsciousness and should try to avoid fully awaking or arousing too much. Try not to turn on bright lights. For this reason, a nightlight in the rest room is a good idea. Keeping it as dark as possible, attempt to make it to the rest room and return to bed quickly, so hopefully you will be able to get back to sleep. Often, you think you are fully awake, when you are still semiconscious. Don't make the mistake of getting something to eat or turning on the TV, when you should just rest in bed and see if sleep will ensue.

Perhaps you can't get back to sleep. Just enjoy resting and relish being in the bed quietly. Often, sleep will return before you know it. If not, rest peacefully, and don't get anxious about not sleeping. Think relaxing thoughts of fun things you did as a child or a favorite vacation spot. Send thoughts far away that cause you to worry or work up your adrenaline—relax and rest. Don't stress if you can't go back to sleep—just rest. Even if you don't fully sleep, rest is very beneficial.

One of my favorite guilty pleasures in life is taking a nap. There is nothing more personally satisfying—than going with it—when I feel the need coming over me for a nap. Having the room extra cool and dark, curling up with a luxuriously soft blanket, while slipping into brief but deep sleep, is for me, heaven on earth—especially if I am allowed to wake up naturally, on my own. If you've traveled and suffer jet lag or it's the holidays and you've stayed up too late celebrating or playing Santa, try to catch as many naps as you can.

However, naps do not provide all the benefits that a good night's sleep provides. We need to be in sync with the circadian rhythm of our bodies. Therefore, naps, as delicious as I think they are, do not compensate for chronic insomnia at night.

Circadian rhythm, known as your "internal body clock,"

is a physiological phenomenon that regulates your hormones and sleep patterns against the natural backdrop of the light-dark cycle, in a 24 hour day—based on the rising and setting of the sun. Naps can hamper that cycle. So this is not a permanent solution. Napping is only for the occasion when you are catching up on sleep, due to an overload or disruption in your schedule, rather than true ongoing insomnia (https://en.wikipedia.org/wiki/Circadian_rhythm).

For women, it is no coincidence that the menstrual cycle is 28 days and the cycle of the moon is 28 days. It is good for women; especially women of childbearing years, to sleep near a window. Soaking up moonlight facilitates the rhythm of the 28-day cycle. It keeps the woman in sync with nature, helping her body balance and regulate hormones. So, try to position your bed near a window that receives moonlight. Natural light does not hamper sleep like artificial light does. Just like sun bathing, try moon bathing.

HORMONES AND SLEEP

Menopausal women should consider hormone replacement therapy (HRT). Pellets containing estrogen and testosterone are surgically implanted into the butt cheek, while progesterone is taken by mouth. This hormonal replenishment and balancing act brings the menopausal symptoms that wreak havoc on sleep satiation to a screeching halt—working to assuage all that tossing and turning throughout the night. Hot flashes cause the woman to kick off the covers, followed by residual sweating—most likely leading to shivers—which result in reaching for and pulling up the same covers that were just kicked off. Throughout the night, the woman is hot and cold while fighting with covers, making it impossible to sleep.

If menopause has set in, pajamas and sheets made of 100% cotton are mandatory to survive the night. I love PeachSkin

Sheets. If you are cold, they keep you warm, and if you are hot, they will keep you cool. I highly recommend them. They are incredibly soft but affordable with the feel of 1500 thread count sheets (go to www.peachskinsheets.com).

HRT is controversial, so I recommend starting with the book, *The Hormone Cure*, by Sara Gottfried, MD. This can help you decide what your best course of action might be for balancing your hormones and managing those pesky hot flashes.

It is far better to replenish and balance hormones through diet and lifestyle change. For example, the overall calming effect of progesterone cream is a viable option in balancing hormones, when implemented in conjunction with a healthy diet.

Applying progesterone cream before retreating for the day can act as a sleep aid. Make sure you use a pea size portion on your wrist, groin, neck, or places where there is a superficial venous system visible to the naked eye, so that the cream is absorbed into the bloodstream. Rotate these sites to avoid resistance to absorption.

Ridding cigarette smoking from your life and keeping your diet alkaline (by drinking lemon water and vegetable juices), are two other positive choices that will balance hormones for better sleep.

To further promote an alkaline pH in the body, avoid sugary drinks, coffee, alcohol, dairy, meats, and spicy foods. In addition, eat lots of leafy green vegetables, high in calcium, along with edible beans—known to be estrogenic. Apparently, women from Japan have managed to escape the phenomenon known as menopause because of the foods they consume. Menopause hasn't really existed in their culture, but with recent western changes in their diet, menopause is becoming more of an issue. The way the Japanese traditionally eat and live automatically keeps the thyroid, cortisol, and estrogen hormones more balanced. Research the Japanese diet. Eat as closely to their way of eating as possible and see if you don't sleep much better. (Diet will be discussed further in the N section: Nutrition.) (www.pcrm.org/health/health-topics/a-natural-approach-to-menopause).

The sad paradox is that estrogen tends to increase if melatonin decreases. This has been linked to both prostate and breast cancer. Both of these type cancers are due to an increase in the bad estrogens that are circulating throughout the body. Both are often treated with the same approach (www.every-dayhealth.com/columns/eric-cohen-breathe-well-sleep-well/dangerous-link-between-lack-of-sleep-cancer/).

THE PROSTATE AND SLEEP

Doctors tell us, if men live long enough, they will eventually develop prostate cancer. Our lifestyle choices make this much more probable than it needs to be. Microwaves and plastic containers, to name a few culprits, cause leaching of plastic and bad estrogens to compromise the prostate, even more than the natural aging process already does. As the prostate ages, it begins to enlarge over time, adversely affecting the man's ability to hold his urine at night. (www.everydayhealth.com/mens-health/enlarged-prostate.aspx).

Men that suffer from a loss of sleep, as a result of getting up and urinating throughout the night, need to limit liquids before going to bed. Drink your water throughout the day before 7 p.m., and that will help significantly. Think about it. If you are getting up throughout the night to urinate, your mind will never fully rest. Your dreams will be hampered and restorative sleep will not occur.

SLEEP AND RELATED BREATHING MALADIES

Sleep loves a quiet mind. It may help to hush your mind, if you concentrate on your breathing. Inhaling and exhaling can help lull you to sleep. The in and out breathing sensation, if truly focused on, can prepare the mind for sleep. Perhaps this breathing action can act as a lullaby for insomniacs. The more you practice this maneuver, the more effective this little technique becomes (more on quieting the mind in the U section: Uncluttering Your Mind) (www.drweil.com/drw/u/ART00521/three-breathing-exercises.html).

Just like frequent urination is a sleep robber, sleep apnea is a condition where sleep is interrupted. Most often, but not always, this disorder is accompanied by snoring, followed by brief to long periods of silence, appearing that the person is not breathing. With this condition, frequently it is reported that headaches are experienced on awakening, and are accompanied by a dry, sore throat in the morning. If not addressed, sleep apnea can lead to even more serious problems, such as, congestive heart failure and hypothyroidism. If you are concerned that you, or someone you love, may have this problem, it is very important to have a sleep study performed to determine if there is any cause for concern.

Perhaps you have seen this in another person, or someone has told you they've observed you while sleeping, and they are concerned that you demonstrate some of these breathing patterns. Recently, I met a lovely lady who learned she needed her tonsils removed. Her daughter was observing her sleep and realized her mother really couldn't breathe. Consequently, she was not completely sleeping. Katherine went to her ENT and discovered she needed her tonsils removed, because they were enormous. This was hampering her breathing, causing her to lose precious sleep. She was always exhausted but with good reason. A tonsillectomy gave her a new lease on life.

Now, many of the hospitals have sleep disorders centers, with state of the art sleep labs. Check with your doctor or call these hospital units to see if you qualify for a sleep study. Many times, you can go to the sleep center and pick up equipment that allows you to conduct the sleep study from the comfort of your own home. Go online, if you can't get to a hospital, and review the options available for in-home sleep studies. Prices vary widely, depending on the equipment you choose.

The Mayo Clinic defines and outlines the various types of sleep apnea:

Sleep apnea is a potentially serious sleep disorder, whereby breathing repeatedly stops and starts. You or a loved one may have sleep apnea, if you snore loudly and feel tired—even after a full night's sleep.

The main types of sleep apnea are:

- Obstructive sleep apnea—the more common form that occurs when throat muscles relax.

- Central sleep apnea—occurs when your brain doesn't send proper signals to the muscles that control breathing.

- Complex sleep apnea syndrome—also known as Treatment-emergent central sleep apnea—occurs when someone has both obstructive sleep apnea and central sleep apnea.

There are at least two breathing devices for this condition— the C-pap and the Bi-pap—as well as other mouthpieces. Becoming more fit and losing abdominal fat can help, if not completely alleviate, some of the problems that require the use of these various breathing aids and equipment. Unfortunately, none of these items are particularly sexy, but they do get the job done. It is encouraging that every day there are new inventions. For example, they finally have a gadget for sleep apnea that claims to eliminate the traditional breathing mask, resembling a deep-sea diver. For more information, go to the American Sleep Association website www.sleepassociation. org.

One such company is Transcend. They have developed a

mini C-pap device that was created with the active, on-the-go person, in mind. It is small, quiet, and travel friendly. Another company, Human Design Medical, helps it's clientele by also increasing the portability of the C-pap machine and reducing the size, so that it is small enough to rest in the palm of your hand.

My most encouraging discovery in the field of sleep apnea is technology from a company called Inspire. They have a battery-operated device that can be surgically implanted in an outpatient setting. You keep a remote control next to your bed. Once you are settled in bed for sleep, you turn on the device. Electrical impulses stimulate the muscles behind the tongue to keep your breathing pathway open. Therefore, you eliminate the obstruction your own anatomy creates. This is a much more appealing, as well as, sexier approach to offsetting sleep apnea for those with this debilitating condition. For more information, visit the Inspire website(www.inspiresleep. com/what-is-inspire-therapy/how-inspire-therapy-works/).

THE SEXY SIDE OF SLEEP

Speaking of sexy, the research is in. Couples that practice sex are more orgasmic when both participants are properly prepared for a good night's sleep. The release of wonderful hormones produces an "oxytocin" effect, facilitating a more balanced ensemble of cortisol and sex hormones—the perfect set up for mutually sound sleep to ensue. We've already concluded that people who get enough sleep have an easier time losing belly fat, which in turn, benefits a couple's sex life. When everything is in place for a healthy "sleep" life, chances are a healthier sex life will commence, which only contributes to restorative sleep—potentially and hopefully—further enhancing your sex life. What a nice vicious cycle! (http:// mic.com/articles/104290/cuddling-with-your-partner-does-something-very-surprising-to-your-health).

Recalling *Holiday*, our movie, and Amanda once again—the minute she remodels her life, her sleep problems disappear like tear stains in the rain. What does her remodel entail? She is in a bad relationship, but it's because she lives for her job, making her life out of balance. Could it be you too need to remodel your life by looking at your relationships and the roles you are fulfilling? Ask yourself, "What's really keeping me up at night?" Do you need to make a few tweaks and adjustments to your life, or do you need a major overhaul? We will more fully examine this question in the remaining sections of the N.U.R.S.E. Approach to Restorative Sleep.

 ## SLEEP Q-TIPS FOR GETTING YOU AND YOUR KIDS TO BED AT AN EARLIER HOUR:

- Start a family tradition. Instead of setting an alarm clock for morning rises, set an alarm clock for bedtime preparation. You've been warned about computers, televisions, and handheld devices, so let's get serious! Even if you are single and live alone, consider setting an alarm as a reminder to prepare for bed.

- Make night time rituals a fun time where everyone has a snack that produces sleep, such as a bite of banana with some almond butter. (It's so good and good for you.)

- Have a family time where everyone says one thing they are thankful for that day, as you tuck them in for the night. If you are single or live alone keep a gratitude journal next to your bed and every night before sleeping, jot something down from that day that caused you to be grateful.

- You may want to a have a family devotion. There are so many wonderful devotionals. It is one of the single most important gifts you can give yourself and your children. I was blessed to have this growing up and it was life changing—as well as character developing for me. I thank God, even though we gave my dad push back, he was firm. I remember it like it was yesterday. Thank you, Daddy.

- Give the kids points that accumulate each week for brushing their teeth and other night time activities, so they can work toward earning a big treat. Maybe the family can go to Disney World or something smaller, such as their favorite new movie release. You can do something special for yourself, as well. Perhaps you can catch up on your DVRs while you eat your favorite meal. Be creative!

PART II
The N.U.R.S.E. Approach to Restorative Sleep

N: THE N.U.R.S.E. APPROACH TO RESTORATIVE SLEEP:

Nutrition for Sleep Based on Joshua Rosenthal's:
Primary Nutrition
Secondary Nutrition

ROSENTHAL'S PRIMARY NUTRITION

This section deals with the problem of being sleep starved, and the nutrition that can help you start sleeping again. "Sleep is the fuel of life," according to Gayle Green, author of *Insomniacs*, and the blog, *Sleep Starved*. On the subject of sleep, she states, "It's nourishing; it's restorative. And when you are robbed of it, you are really deprived of a basic kind of sustenance."

Jordan Rubin, author of *The Maker's Diet*, wants you to know that quality sleep is so vital, he often refers to it as "the most important non-nutrient you can get."

My role is to coach you to eat in such a way that you maximize the amount of Zzz's you acquire, thereby adequately supplementing your life with this vitally restorative, and rejuvenating non-nutrient—sleep. By now you are clear on one thing. As we continue to track our friend, Amanda—she is not sleeping and you are about to learn what's keeping her up at night. Perhaps, you are dealing with the same root problem.

Primary food, in the truest sense, is your soul food—not the traditional "southern fried, meat-and-three" soul food of the deep south. But rather, food that sustains your mental, willful, and emotional passions.

Joshua Rosenthal, author of *Integrative Nutrition,* taught me, at the Integrative Institute for Nutrition, that primary food is the personal fulfillment you derive from family, friends, relationships, career, physical activity, and spirituality. What you think of as food, in the traditional sense—the stuff you buy at the grocery store, bring home, cook, chew, and swallow—is really secondary food, or your physical nourishment.

I'll bet you can recall being a child busy at play with your friends, enjoying your activity so much that your mom had to call you several times before you surrendered and finally came to the dinner table to eat. You were so satiated with your real passions—playtime and friends—that eating supper was secondary to anything else, even if you needed the nourishment.

By imparting his idea that the food you eat is secondary to the passions that fuel your life, Joshua gave me the insight to move forward with my original N.U.R.S.E. coaching model.

After nursing school, I went for my MA in psychology with an emphasis in counseling. I wanted to combine nutrition, psychology, and holistic nursing, in order to help women overcome autoimmune diseases, brought on by stress and poor nutrition. I had beaten Grave's disease—an autoimmune disease, resulting in hyperthyroidism—by implementing this same, three-pronged, comprehensive model.

However, the Dean of the college was not ready for my unique, three-layered approach to therapy. She strongly advised me to choose nursing, nutrition, or psychology, but counseled me to abandon the idea of combining the three areas of study. "Pick one hat and wear it," she barked.

As a result of this dean's stance, I shelved the N.U.R.S.E. coaching idea—as I have outlined it for you in this book, until I met Joshua Rosenthal. His nutritional concept of primary and secondary food, empowered me to move forward, a decade later, with my N.U.R.S.E. approach to therapy.

Currently, I am able to help men and women conquer disease—just as I did, in overcoming my own battle with Grave's disease, while wearing all three hats—nutrition, psychology, and nursing. Earning my Certification as a Nutrition Coach (CNC), provided the additional expertise, paired with my nursing credentials, to give me a voice in the revolution that's changing the world's current view of smart, healthy food choices.

As you progress with me, on this N.U.R.S.E. acronym journey,

Nutrition

Uncluttering

Remodeling your life

Spirituality

Exercising

the entire R section of *Nurse, Nurse, I'm Worse! Can You Help Me Sleep?* is dedicated to the problems surrounding primary food, possibly causing your sleep issues.

Let's transition for a moment to our character, Amanda, from the movie, *Holiday*. She is beautiful, perfectly fit—with not an ounce of fat on her body. Most likely, this is because she benefits from a California diet, where there's always an ample supply of some of the healthiest food on the planet. No doubt, Amanda has some great genes working in her favor, as well. She also has access to plenty of sunshine, fresh air, and clean water—the perfect environment for physical activity in the outdoors. She looks as though she practices yoga.

So, Amanda is sitting pretty when it comes to secondary nutrition. But what about primary nutrition? Once she takes care of her malnourished soul by improving her primary food, through a remodeled life, she is able to sleep.

Whether it be a person, people, family members, a calling, a dream, or a goal—or a combination of all your passions—what difference does it make, if you eat meticulously and swallow a dozen vitamins everyday—but your life is empty and you're miserable with your choices? You may eat clean, exercise like a fiend, have the perfect arms, and sport the flattest stomach ever, but still be malnourished concerning primary food.

If you are a free person—able to exercise your own will—you are the sum total of all your decisions. Even if you are the victim of a tragedy, you can still decide, in response to the situation, what your attitude will be—good, bad, or indifferent.

Some of the most beautiful, physically fit, disciplined people—the ones that never eat a cookie—are the most disillusioned when it comes to their main relationships and life's work. Are you one of these loved-starved, exhausted, perfect people? If so, you are suffering from primary food deficiency.

I know a woman, just like Amanda, who lives in a perfect body and resides in a charmingly exquisite house, with a to-die-for closet. She is a dynamite cook and is quite the sex kitten. Her exterior world is pristinely coifed, but her primary food pantry is empty.

Life can get messy. And when it does, do you find yourself overcompensating by becoming too controlling with your exterior world? It's okay to try and bring order and beauty to your surroundings, as long as you keep it balanced. Guard against the temptation to control other people.

People should never feel less important to you than your

clean, flawless, house. Make your picture-perfect world a place where imperfect people can still live and laugh, in step with you, as you journey through life. You'll find that this kind of living helps you get rid of those sheep you've been counting at night. You'll get those Zzz's to come around every night, right on time when you surrender perfectionism. I know it's easier said than done!

Perhaps you know people who allow their careers to consume and define them. You may be this kind of person. If so, then know that you are, perchance, the victim of sleep deprivation, as a direct result of being super uptight.

Hopefully, you are not an insomniac control freak—someone who never has nightmares because you're too busy giving other people nightmares—as a result of your own sleep deprivation. Excessive, controlling behaviors often cause people to become insomniacs, and can be the reason you are sleep deprived. Is this you or anyone you know? It is definitely true of our character, Amanda. She's a hot mess when it comes to this aspect of her life. (There is more on this in the R section.)

ROSENTHAL'S SECONDARY NUTRITION

You can now explore with me some ideas in the secondary nutrition department for restorative sleep. But here's a word of caution. The content in this section is quite exhaustive—in more ways than one. Most of this information is not for night reading, unless you are looking for something to put you to sleep—and since that just happens to be the case—knock yourself out, literally. However, I do want you to actually retain what you are reading. This is "need-to-know" information.

Perhaps you should save the following reading material for when you're enjoying your morning coffee or preparing your grocery list. You can more readily absorb this compilation once you are rested and rejuvenated for the new day. By incorporating these dietary suggestions into your daily food choices, the goal is to help you experience restorative sleep. This portion of the Nutrition section will act as a resource guide that you will refer to often.

My own coaching model—the N.U.R.S.E. Approach to Restorative Sleep—is designed to concentrate solely on nutrition that helps you sleep. Therefore, for the purpose of this section, this is not an all-inclusive overview of nutrition, but this material is limited to foods that maximize your ability to enjoy restorative sleep.

There are so many books about nutrition. You can easily find one for any and every possible aspect of nutrition. I highly recommend Jordan Rubin's book, *The Maker's Diet,* as a comprehensive, go-to book for your overall nutritional needs. In general, a healthy diet for the waking portion of the day also carries over to what is healthy for the sleeping portion of the 24-hour cycle.

Food, nourishment, and the various aspects of "eating" are deeply woven into your everyday thinking and conversation, but I'll bet you've never realized to what extent. Have you ever stopped to think of how many times you refer to food in your daily conversations? Think of all the food clichés. Here are just a few, but you may come up with more of your own:

• You are what you eat.

• An apple a day keeps the doctor away.

• If you can't take the heat, stay out of the kitchen.

• That's the way the old cookie crumbles.

• He got caught with his hand in the cookie jar.

• Life's not a bowl full of cherries.

• Life is like a box of chocolates.

• It's as easy as pie.

- It's a piece of cake.
- That's just icing on the cake.
- You can't have your cake and eat it too.
- She's cool as a cucumber.
- There are no free meals in life.
- I'm done. Stick a fork in it!
- Now you're cooking with gas!
- You catch more flies with honey than with vinegar.
- Make your words sweet because one day, you may have to eat them.
- He still has some sour grapes over my promotion.
- I'd love to give him a knuckle sandwich.
- Here comes the big cheese.
- Who cut the cheese?
- He dropped the subject like a hot potato.
- The proof is in the pudding.
- I'm tired of working for peanuts.
- Eat your heart out!
- That's just peachy!
- Bring home the bacon.
- It will sell like hotcakes.
- He earned some brownie points today.
- She was trying to butter him up.
- He's my bread and butter.
- He "souped up" the engine.
- She's a nut.

- He's nuttier than a fruitcake.
- That kid is a couch potato.
- I smell something fishy.
- Why is she crying over spilt milk?
- Don't put all your eggs in one basket.

These are just a few examples of food clichés that are used in our conversations day in and day out. And the list goes on . . . Can you think of some of your own?

_____

_____

_____

_____

_____

_____

_____

Your words tell all. Listen to what you and others are saying. The very essence of who you are is related to what you "feed on." This is not just in reference to what you ingest physically, but also mentally, emotionally, and spiritually.

Every person is unique, and researchers are finding that nutritional choices and plans are "bio-individual"—a term I learned from Joshua Rosenthal. He teaches that "one man's food, is another man's poison." So, what works for you may not work for someone else. Find books that are specific to your unique nutritional needs and come up with your own plan.

In forging your bio-individual path to sound nutrition—and your overall health—you have to apply wisdom and diligence. For example, you've probably heard that a warm glass of milk will help you become sleepy. Perhaps you can drink milk and even enjoy dairy products—without any allergic reaction—especially if you are a B-blood type. But someone else might be adversely affected by dairy, due to lactose intolerance.

For all of you lactose-intolerant people—about 29 million Americans—you might want to consider the more likely problem of pasteurization, a process of heating milk to prevent potential contamination of microorganisms, such as Salmonella, E. coli, and Listeria. Most of the milk you drink is heated to 280°. Low pasteurized milk—heating milk to 145°—is the closest thing to raw milk you can purchase in most of the United States.

Only eight states allow raw milk to be sold in the stores for human consumption: Arizona, California, Connecticut, Maine, Pennsylvania, South Carolina, New Mexico, and Washington. I live in Georgia, where you can buy raw milk at Red Bandana—but it is marked "pet food." Why is this an issue? Because 85% of people with lactose intolerance can tolerate raw milk.

Pasteurization destroys the wonderful benefits of milk, the healthy fats, protein, vitamins, and enzymes—all for the sake of killing potentially harmful bacteria. Despite the fact that milk is at the bottom of the list, when compared to all food-borne illnesses from produce—poultry, eggs, beef, and even seafood—it still is singled out for criticism. For perspective, consider that from 1990 to 2006 only 315—1.3% of all 24,000 reported food-borne illnesses came from dairy products.

Pasteurized milk turns rancid, if it spoils, but raw milk simply sours. Pasteurized milk is difficult to digest, but raw milk is one of the most perfect foods you can ingest (from the 2015 Raw Milk Symposium, "Why Raw Milk?", Sally Fallon, MA).

According to Paul McKenna, writing in, *I Can Make You Sleep,* milk contains tryptophan, "the magic sleep chemical." But if you don't like milk or can't drink it—never fear. McKenna tells you that eating a normal healthy diet contains more than adequate amounts of tryptophan, which will benefit your ability to sleep. Here is a list of other foods containing significant amounts of tryptophan:

- Yogurt
- Fish
- Poultry
- Eggs
- Red meat
- Bananas
- Mangoes
- Turkey—infamous for causing you to nap after eating Thanksgiving dinner

In fact, tryptophan is so plentiful that you would have to go to great lengths to avoid consuming the needed amount in your diet.

According to Peter J. D' Adamo, ND, of all the blood types, A-blood types do better with a vegetarian diet. Although controversial, the premise of Adamo's book, *Eat Right for Your Type*, is based on the idea that different blood types require different diets. This idea supports, the concept of bio-individuality, when it comes to personal diets.

First and foremost, no matter what your blood type, the universal mandate for good sound nutrition is to eat fresh foods, seasonal foods, and locally grown foods. Not every food has to be organic, but there are some foods that do need to be organic, due to the enormous amount of pesticides used to grow them. Pay attention to which organic foods are a must for you. Some foods typically have a lower pesticide load and, as a result, are less contaminated. This means they don't have to be organic.

Here is a list of the "dirty dozen," plus a few others, that need to be organic:

- Peaches
- Nectarines
- Strawberries
- Grapes
- Celery
- Spinach
- Sweet bell peppers
- Cucumbers
- Cherry tomatoes
- Snap peas, imported
- Potatoes
- Hot peppers
- Kale
- Collard greens

Here is the list of the clean fifteen that don't have to be organic (www.drweil.com/drw/u/ART02984/Foods-You-Dont-Have-to-Buy-Organic.html):

- Avocados
- Sweet corn
- Pineapples
- Cabbage
- Sweet peas (frozen)
- Onions
- Asparagus

- Mangoes

- Papayas

- Kiwi

- Eggplant

- Grapefruit

- Cantaloupe (domestic)

- Cauliflower

- Sweet potatoes

Why is this so important? Chemicals affect hormones and digestion. You have to pay close attention to how these chemicals react with your body chemistry.

Certain foods processed with preservatives and additives can wreak havoc on your hormones. They can trigger hot flashes, if you are peri-menopausal or menopausal, causing you to toss and turn all night. For the most part, avoid anything in a bag or a package—potato chips, crackers, or cookies. Packaged foods of all types, such as, frozen dinners, are filled with preservatives and additives—vicious enemies of your hormones.

If you can't pronounce the ingredients, you probably shouldn't eat them. It is a good rule of thumb to avoid food from the middle aisles. It's inferior to the fresh food along the outer edges of the grocery store. When you shop, purchase fresh produce, meat, eggs, poultry, milk, and other dairy products. Avoid processed meats, as well as deli and sandwich meats because of sodium nitrites—a possible carcinogen.

Foods that are white—crackers, popcorn, rice, potatoes, floury foods, to name a few—convert to another culprit, sugar. Even milk needs to be monitored, because lactose is a sugar. Sugar is an inflammatory food causing blood sugars to spike, resulting in inflammation. It should be coupled with fat and protein to prevent blood glucose from skyrocketing. That is why whole milk is better for you than milk with reduced fat.

Inflammation will cause joints to hurt, keeping you awake at night. If you have too much sugar before bed, your body will convince you to urinate during the night to get rid of some of the excess sugar in your system. To learn more about the role of inflammation in your body, and how to prevent it by eating correctly, read Barry Sears' book, *The Zone*.

Sally Fallon Morell is an advocate for eating a healthy traditional diet. Her work and website, www.westonaprice.org/about-the-foundation/about-us, are profoundly eye-opening. To learn more about your food and how it is being compromised, even altered, go to her website to visit the Weston A. Price Foundation: Wise Traditions in Food, Farming and the Healing Arts. You can discover the changes that have occurred throughout the years, to our food from the early 1900s until our current food processes—and not necessarily changes for the better. Don't gamble with your food by ingesting milk from cloned animals and eating plant foods that are genetically modified. These are just a few of the things you will be astonished to learn about your food at this website.

The food you and I consume is not the same food our grandparents enjoyed. We have all been told many lies about what is good for us and what is not. I explored this matter, by focusing earlier on milk, because it is known that a warm glass of milk helps you fall asleep. However, there is so much controversy surrounding the pros and cons of drinking milk. I find that it is the perfect example of all that is going on adversely with our food—politically, nutritionally, and agriculturally.

For instance, the United States is the only industrialized nation that approves genetically modified milk. Almost all of the other nations do not allow this. Look for labels on milk to see if they use rBGH—a hormone that has been linked to increased risks for certain cancers. Unfortunately, the FDA has also approved cloned milk. If you are able, try to buy organic milk.

The use of rBGH or rBST causes the cow to produce much more milk than she normally would. With the excessive milk production, the udders are overused and frequently the mammary glands become infected. The cow is then given antibiotics, which is passed on to you and me, if we drink the milk. Overuse of antibiotics in treating the cow can cause them to become ineffective in conquering infectious bacterial growth. These awful infections yield terrible pain and discomfort to the poor animal, not to mention the pus that ends up in the milk. This is becoming increasingly prevalent and is becoming common practice.

I applaud Sally Fallon Morell for her activist voice concerning the importance of nutrient-dense foods. For more information with other foods besides milk, check out two books by Sally, *Nourishing Traditions*, and *Eat Fat, Lose Fat*.

Getting back to basics is the challenge of the day. Frequently, in the food department, what's keeping you up at night is not the food itself. It's what is being done to the food. Before you purchase food, pay attention to the labels, which describe the process your food has undergone—it's important.

These are the labels to look for and what they mean:

Antibiotic-Free—No antibiotics were given during the animal's lifetime. Raised without antibiotics. This is important because you are what you eat, and society, as a whole, is building up a resistance to antibiotics because of overuse. You can reach a point where antibiotics don't work for you. Excessive use of antibiotics has been linked to cancer because this practice weakens the immune system. You need a strong immune system to ward off budding cancer cells throughout the body. Although you may never know it, at any given time, you can have cancer cells, but if you are healthy, your body will destroy them before they start growing and spreading.

Cage-Free—This only means no cages, but most likely raised in overcrowded, poor, indoor conditions. Look for pastured or pasture-raised.

Fair-Trade—Farmers and workers received a fair wage and worked in acceptable conditions throughout the growing and packaging process.

Free-Range or Free-Roaming—Only defined by the USDA for egg and poultry production. This label applies as long as the producer allows the birds to have outside privileges and to engage in normal behaviors. This does not mean cruelty-free, antibiotic-free, or that the fowl has spent most of its time outdoors.

GMO-Free, Non-GMO, or No GMOs—Foods not derived from genetically modified organisms. This label does not encompass animals or plants—genetically engineered from the DNA of bacteria, viruses, or other plants and animals.

Grain-Fed—Look for 100% vegetarian diet with no animal by-products.

Grass-Fed/Grass Finished—The animal was fed grass, its natural diet. The animal was not fed grain, animal by-products, synthetic hormones, or antibiotics to promote or prevent disease. Antibiotics were reserved for use of treating actual disease. This is not very comforting after learning about over-stimulating the cow's milk production with the use of rBGH, resulting in infections from over using the cows udders. Look for "grass finished" to ensure the animal was grass-fed at the feed lot before slaughter.

Healthy—Must be low in saturated fat and contain low amounts of cholesterol and sodium. Certain foods must contain at least 10% of these nutrients: vitamins A and C, iron, calcium, protein, and fiber.

Heritage—These animals are valued for their rich taste. Often, they contain a higher fat content than commercial breeds. Heritage farmers use sustainable production methods, saving the animal from extinction, preserving genetic diversity.

Hormone-Free—Legally, hogs and poultry cannot be given hormones. If there are no labels on the meat you are purchasing, ask your butcher if it is hormone-free. The USDA has banned the term "hormone-free," but animals that were raised without added growth hormones can be labeled "no added hormones."

Natural—No artificial color, flavors, preservatives, or other artificial ingredients. This simply means there was minimal processing of meats and poultry. This label is inferior because it does not necessarily mean sustainable, organic, humanely raised, and free of antibiotics and hormones.

Nonirradiated—The food has not been exposed to radiation to kill disease-causing bacteria. No testing has been done to know if irradiated food is safe for human consumption.

Pasture-Raised—Animals were able to move around freely in their natural habitat and carry out natural habits. Healthier animals result in better meat. This label is similar to grass-fed. It clearly indicates the animal was raised outdoors on a pasture.

rBGH-Free or rBST-Free—This hormone is approved by the FDA, but is not approved for the European Union, Canada, and other industrialized nations. This hormone—recombinant bovine growth hormone or recombinant bovine somatotropin—is a genetically engineered growth hormone injected into dairy cows to artificially increase their growth. Remember that this hormone has been linked to certain cancers. Always look to make sure your dairy says rBGH-free or rBST-free.

Organic—The USDA has about eight guidelines for agricultural farms, concerning the labels for its products. These must be followed to the letter and be verified by a USDA-approved independent agency.

-Abstain from application of synthetic fertilizers, pesticides, and sewage sludge for three years prior to certification and then continually throughout their organic license.

- No use of genetically modified organisms and no irradiation.

- Implement positive soil building, conservation, manure management, and crop rotation practices.

- Allow outdoor access and pasture for livestock.

- Refrain from antibiotic and hormone use in animals.

- Sustains animals on 100% organic feed.

- Avoid contamination during the processing of organic products.

- Keep records of all operations.

In order for a food to receive the USDA Organic seal, 95%–100% of its ingredients are organic. Organic foods can have no hydrogenated or trans fats. In order to advertise on the front panel, the food must be 70%–95% organic, but if less than 70% organic, then this is how it must be advertised on the side panel (adapted from: www.sustainabletable.org/944/these-labels-are-so-confusing).

Hippocrates told us centuries ago: "Let food be thy medicine and medicine be thy food." If you eat right and take care of yourself, you shouldn't need a sleeping pill or a pharmaceutical intervention. I am not an advocate of medicine, except as a last resort. So, I will not address sleep medications, except to mention crisis intervention for severe anxiety and depression.

You will never sleep optimally if you are taking sleep medication. If you are experiencing insomnia due to clinical depression, however—or some other malady related to sleep and anxiety—you may have to be on meds for a season to resolve the matter.

A classic symptom of major depression is waking up at 3:00 or 4:00 in the morning and not being able to go back to sleep for more than a night or two. Once depression is treated with the appropriate meds, early morning awakenings are often alleviated. The goal is always to wean you off the meds eventually, but under medical supervision. This information is based on ideas from, Daniel Kripke, *The Dark Side of Sleeping Pills*.

I have a friend who had a car accident and suffered a traumatic brain injury, resulting in severe insomnia. Medical supervision and intense pharmacological intervention was required to induce sleep. She did not sleep at all for almost a week. Situations like hers are rare and are the exception to "the-no-medication" rule I favor. However, each individual situation must be considered, including your own unique set of circumstances. Sometimes, pharmacology is a must, especially with depression and anxiety—at least for a season.

Serotonin is an endorphin that plays a huge role in mood disorders and sleep. There are occasions where sleep is so compromised that pharmaceuticals can be a great help, but only under a doctor's care. The quality of sleep will still be a compromised version of ideal sleep, though—compared to what you would have if you did not take pills. Medication is a two-faced friend. You may doze off with it, but the ability to sleep is inferior to naturally induced sleep. Pharmacological intervention hampers true, deep, and restorative sleep.

You have to make up your own mind to educate yourself about your choices of medication. Again, let food be your medicine, when it comes to sleep. Remember, you are what you eat, which also plays a role in how well you sleep.

Supplements can be just as bad as pharmaceuticals. For example, melatonin supplements are often made from cow urine and all kinds of toxic fillers. The truth is that you can't be certain of what you are taking, unless the supplements are 100% non-GMO plant-based. When it comes to melatonin, it's best for you to eat foods that increase the naturally occurring melatonin in your body, rather than popping a pill. Plus, your body can build a tolerance to melatonin supplements, and then you are really in a pickle—another food cliché!

Melatonin, the sleep-inducing hormone that regulates your circadian rhythm, can be found in these foods—making them excellent choices for a bed time snack, but only in small quantities (www.onegreenplanet.org/.../foods-that-help-produce-melatonin-oats-bananas -and-more/):

(1) Bananas—contain magnesium, vitamin B6, and natural complex carbs. These nutrients, along with tryptophan—an amino acid—produce serotonin, promoting relaxation.

(2) Oats—I love a bowl of oatmeal in the morning, but you might want to consider eating oatmeal in the evening. Oats are loaded with an assortment of beneficial vitamins and minerals that not only carry you off to sleepy town, but they also regulate your sleep throughout the night.

(3) Pineapple is a great fruit. Because of its digestive properties, you can combine it, as an option, with any meal. Pineapples have more melatonin-boosting benefits than bananas or oats.

(4) Oranges—are delicious. Due to their vitamin C content, along with calcium and B vitamins, oranges help you produce melatonin more efficiently.

(5) Cherries—are a melatonin-producing powerhouse.

They also fight inflammation in the body, which can reduce joint pain, resulting in better sleep. Cherries may also help you sleep longer. They are so rich in nourishment, they create quality melatonin in the body.

(6) Walnuts—are another fabulous choice of food that helps promote the synthesis of melatonin.

Valerian root is an herb that promotes sleep. If it takes you forever to fall asleep—followed by waking up, on and off, throughout the night—try valerian root. This natural sedative works to increase your overall ability to drift off to sleep and stay asleep, improving the quality and quantity of your sleep. A secondary effect of this herb is that it is very calming to your mild anxieties, thereby decreasing nervousness.

Rose hip is packed full of Vitamin C, which works to repair the body while you sleep, especially collagen. You've heard of needing beauty sleep; well this ingredient helps you acquire some of the best beauty sleep around.

Vitamin B complexes, found in food, are the anti-stress vitamins. These vitamins are busy, working to decrease nervousness, as well as helping your hair shine, skin glow, nails become stronger, eyes sparkle, and liver hum.

B vitamins give you energy, while they partner with melatonin to regulate the sleep–wake cycle. They also act with serotonin and norepinephrine to improve your mood. Most meats and fish have vitamin B6. Plant foods such as sweet potatoes, potatoes, bananas, winter squash, broccoli, brussel sprouts, and collard greens are rich sources of vitamin B6. Meat, fish, dairy, and eggs supply vitamin B12.

Magnesium and other minerals, such as calcium, are helpful in promoting sleep—as well as other natural remedies—namely, melatonin. Although calcium helps you fall asleep, it cannot be absorbed without adequate amounts of magnesium. Therefore, most calcium tablets have magnesium added, so look for that on the supplement packaging. It's better, however, to eat foods high in magnesium and calcium, such as green leafy vegetables, spinach, kale, and various nuts.

Not to be forgotten is vitamin D. So much is being discovered about vitamin D deficiencies. Most people are lucky if they are getting the recommended daily intake. Some researchers are now saying you may need as much as 10,000 IU per day. The body, if healthy, utilizes 3000–5000 IU per day, but the US Government recommended upper intake level (UL) for vitamin D is set at 4000 IU per day. It is best to have a blood test and see where your levels are and go from there.

The interesting finding is that you should not take vitamin D at night because it works against your melatonin (www.gwern.net/Zeo). The inverse relationship makes it mandatory to take vitamin D in the morning. You will enjoy better REM sleep and wake up in a better mood (refer to www.ncbi.nlm.nih.gov/pubmed/22583560 and www.webmd.com/a-to-z-guides/discomfort-15/better-sleep/slideshow-sleep-tips).

The amount of vitamin D you get from exposing your bare skin to the sun depends on:

- The time of day—your skin produces more vitamin D if you expose it during the middle of the day.

- Where you live—the closer to the equator you live, the easier it is for you to produce vitamin D from sunlight all year round.

- The color of your skin—pale skins make vitamin D more quickly than darker skins.

- The amount of skin you expose—the more skin you expose, the more vitamin D your body will produce.

(www.vitamindcouncil.org/about-vitamin-d/how-do-i-get-the-vitamin-d-my-body-needs)

Now that you have explored, from a secondary nutrition perspective, some foundational sleep inducing foods and nutrients, remember there is also, a primary food aspect to insomnia. Remember primary food is the fuel that feeds and sustains your mental, willful, and emotional passions.

The entire R section of *Nurse, Nurse, I'm Worse! Can You Help Me Sleep?* is dedicated to resolving any potential problems surrounding primary food, possibly causing your sleep issues. In the R section, you'll get a chance to explore the five pillars of rest: (1) residence, (2) resources, (3) roles, (4) relationships, and (5) religion, all of which comprise primary food. But first, let's do some "uncluttering" in the next section, after reviewing a few sleep Q-tips.

 SLEEP Q-TIPS:

- Drink chamomile tea. And if you like it sweetened, use a touch of lavender honey. (You might want to pass on this one if you are prone to frequent night-time urination.)

- Honey, the experts claim, burns fat while you sleep. But less is more because it is sweeter than sugar and has more calories than sugar (www.benefits-of-honey.com).

- Avoid too much sugar at night. Many times urination at night is the body's mechanism to rid itself of excess sugar.

- Lavender scents that are packaged in a variety of forms (such as candles) can promote sleep—but you must put out candles before the final doze!

- Avoid too much caffeine. No caffeine is ideal, but that's not practical. One cup is fine in the early am, but no more than two cups—and no later than 10 a.m.

- During the holidays, special occasions or on weekends, if you want a cup of coffee in the evening, there is a new truly decaffeinated coffee: The Counting Sheep Coffee ($12 at amazon.com) contains valerian, an herb that promotes sleep. So many decaf coffees are known to have as much as 20 mg of caffeine, but not this one (https://www.yahoo.com/health/20-things-you-shouldnt-do-before-bed-113344981198.html).

- Resort to sleep medication only as a last option. Sleep will never be as deep and restorative if it is chemically induced. Using a sleep aid on rare occasions will not be habit forming. However, chronic use of sleep medication will allow your own internal sleep mechanism to become lazy and your quality of sleep will be compromised. You will never reach deep, healing, and restorative sleep, and the ability to dream will be hampered.

- People doze off, on average, 30 to 40 minutes after taking iChill Natural Liquid Sleep Aid, developed to help people relax and "chill" at the end of a long, hard day. This naturally refreshing sleep aid consists of a blend of melatonin, Valerian root, Rose Hips, and B vitamins. Plus, there's an added bonus of no calories and no carbs (http://ichill.com/how-ichill-works).

- Caution: I still prefer eating foods that help your body create your own melatonin. Why? Because often melatonin in a bottle comes from synthetic manmade melatonin, which is identical to the naturally occurring hormone—from bovine brain and urine. You just don't know. Remember Mad Cow disease? Let food be thy medicine. Get your melatonin from non-GMO plant-based foods (http://www.sleeppassport.com/melatonin-supplements.html).

- A great bedtime snack is pureed, slightly chilled bananas and cherries with a touch of vanilla. It's as delicious as a bowl of ice cream and will help you increase your melatonin naturally.

- Nuts and seeds raise serotonin levels and promote relaxation. Keep these in the house for late night snacks: walnuts, almonds, sesame seeds, and pumpkin seeds. Peanuts (legumes) are good, too.

- Avoid these foods before bed—caffeine, not just in coffee, but even in cocoa and green tea, as well. Skip the spicy, heavy foods that keep you awake.

- Oranges—feast on delicious red blood oranges (when in season) for a divine bedtime snack. Eat your fruit, but don't drink the fruit juices. They are too sugary in juice form.

- Nut-butters, spread on small slices of bananas, are a yummy bedtime snack. I love to pair almond butter with bananas. It's crack cocaine for me!

- Tomatoes are a fabulous source of nutrients that produce melatonin naturally. Have a cup of fresh, home-made tomato soup on a cold winter night and doze right off to sleep.

- Try oatmeal—not sweet but savory—for a dinner dish (www.onegreenplanet.org/vegan-food/ways-to-go-savory-with-oatmeal).

U: THE N.U.R.S.E. APPROACH TO RESTORATIVE SLEEP:

Uncluttering—Your Bedroom for Sleep
Create a sanctuary for sleep as a benediction to your day

Uncluttering—Your Mind for Sleep
Rituals and associations for inducing rest

Uncluttering—Your Heart for Sleep
Resolving anger with your bedroom partner
Untangling the soul ties that keep you awake

UNCLUTTERING YOUR BEDROOM FOR SLEEP

Don't you love walking into a beautiful hotel room that is immaculate? That first minute when you open the door, before you unpack, or pull the bed covers back—for a split second, the world stands still. Think about that "Calgon take me away" feeling and why this moment is so soothing. At last, you've escaped the taxing, loud world. You can finally collapse, in your perfect little retreat. But beyond all of that, at least, in the initial moment of entry, the room is clutter-free—regardless of any clutter you may eventually create—you will only find items in the room that are beautiful, useful, and purposeful.

Now consider your own bedroom. What is the ambiance? Does your bedroom whisper a-come-hither invitation to, "Forget the world, leave it all behind, come and dream, rejuvenate—rest?"

Your bedroom should be a sanctuary for sleep. If it's not, then let's get started. Just like the hotel room, if anything in the room is not purposeful, useful, or beautiful, remove it.

The curtains in a hotel room are heavy, thick, and lined with white, for completely darkening the room. Sheers are hung to block out city lights for a muted darkness in the evening, and to ward off heat from sunlight when the shades are open during the day. Take a clue from this scenario. Examine your window treatments. Do they serve you well in the sleep department, helping you get your needed Zzz's?

Look at Amanda's bedroom. It's as great as, or better than, the finest hotel room. Think of every detail she chose to enhance sleep—from the monochromatic muted colors, down to the remote controlled window shades for darkening the room. Who couldn't get their Zzz's in this perfect-for-sleep bedroom? Obviously, Amanda couldn't. However, at least, with a sleep sanctuary like this, she knows how to roll out the red carpet for sleep—once it actually comes around again.

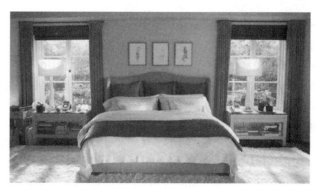

Amanda needs to remodel her life in order to sleep, but definitely not her bedroom. I want your bedroom to be a retreat for sleep. So, look around your bedroom and make an honest assessment. If correcting your bedroom is the only remodeling required to resolve your sleep issues, you'll be able to once again enjoy deep restorative sleep and live optimally.

In 2011, WebMD reported on a study that was conducted by the National Sleep Foundation. Observe this direct quote from David Cloud, NSF Chief Operating Officer, "We've looked a lot at how medical and behavioral issues affect sleep, but we really hadn't looked at the sleep environment in such depth. Frankly, we were surprised to see that senses like touch, feel, and smell were so important."

Really? It's a no brainer. If you have soft, clean sheets that smell fresh and are not scratchy or of a poor quality, you don't need a survey to tell you what you already know. You'll have less distractions and be more comfortable. Therefore, you have a better chance of sleeping, as well as sleeping longer, according to the survey. So vacuum your bedroom and dust it thoroughly, including any ceiling fans or floor fans. As an added bonus, sprinkle a touch of baby powder on your sheets. See if that is not an invitation to snooze that you can't refuse.

This same study revealed that making your bed every day helps you sleep better. In this study, a sample of 1500 randomly selected U.S. participants (ages 25 to 55) revealed they slept great—either every night or almost every night. This was less than half (42%) of the total number surveyed. Of the 1500 sampled, seven out of ten made their bed almost every day, with 19% reporting better sleep.

Along with this finding, I am reminded of a woman who taught me to respect money, using a similar logic. The idea is when you acquire dollar bills, arrange them in your billfold with the faces of the Presidents on top and flatten out all the corners and wrinkles. Stack the bills in your wallet in ascending order of value. Show your money respect and you will change your attitude towards money, supposedly, attracting more of it. Apply that same thought process to sleep. Show sleep a little respect—make your bed every day and create a special welcoming for your long-awaited, fair-weathered friend. See for yourself if sleep doesn't surprise you, by taking up permanent residence in your new sleep friendly bedroom.

Get rid of your lumpy mattress or pillows that have lost their form. Buy the best you can afford. Invest in good linens, comforters, pillows, and mattresses. You owe it to yourself to splurge on the bedroom. It is the most important room in the house. After all the information you've received about the importance of sleep, thus far, I hope you agree. You spend one third of your life sleeping—if you are getting eight hours of sleep per night. And after all, that is the goal.

Some people would argue that the kitchen is the most important room in the house. But if you think about it, chances are, you eat out at least, once or twice a week. Conversely, you probably don't stay in a hotel and sleep away from your house once or twice a week—unless you travel with your job. You and I, most likely, come home to sleep every night (or day if you're doing shift work), during a normal workday week. You can find a place to eat every day, but a place to sleep is a bit more intimate. You are probably spending the benediction of your day in your own bedroom.

The room should be calm and inviting—not too busy or overpowering, reflecting a mutually agreed upon decor between you and your bedroom partner. A bedroom should be muted and soft without being excessively feminine. Appropriate lighting for reading is in order, but no harsh lights are needed in the bedroom—rather, soft light bulbs with a pink hue, for camouflaging skin imperfections. The most conducive surroundings for sleep are void of mirrors and electrical devices. I advocate no TV in the bedroom.

The temperature should be on the cool side. Researchers say the best temperature for a couple is 65.5°, but there should be plenty of covers for the cold natured. It is best if each partner has their own blanket so the two of you are not pulling and tugging the covers throughout the night (http://well.blogs.nytimes.com/2014/07/17/lets-cool-it-in-the-bedroom/?_r=0).

UNCLUTTERING YOUR MIND FOR SLEEP

Now that you have uncluttered your bedroom, let's look at uncluttering your mind so sleep will ensue. When it comes to uncluttering your mind, that's considered a more ethereal aspect of inducing somnolence—the state of being drowsy, or sleepiness. The goal is to reach a deep sense of calm—a state of mind that equates to peace.

Have you ever noticed that thoughts are louder in the dark? Vivian (played by Julia Roberts) from the movie *Pretty Woman*, asks Edward (played by Richard Gere), *"The bad stuff is easier to believe, ever notice that?"* At night, the words that people use to put you down and shame you, or the endless list of things you worry about, come out, and shout at you.

Sadly, the following scenario plays out in millions of homes around the globe every night:

As much as you are loving the television show, you've been nodding off throughout the entire, past half-hour of the episode. You can't imagine anything but passing out, once you get in bed.

Now that you've actually made it to bed, you're under the covers, the lights are out, and you are finally dozing off. When out of the blue, it's as though someone splashes cold water on your face—your mind does a number on you. A million thoughts race through your mind at the speed of light,

"Did I pay the mortgage?"

"I hope he doesn't want that report first thing in the morning!"

"Why does she hate me so much?"

"I wonder if the tires will last another month!"

"Oh, no, I forgot Sara's birthday!"

Suddenly, wanting to sleep more than anything—you find yourself wide awake. Believe it or not, you can train yourself to shut those thoughts down.

Here are a few quick suggestions:

The mind is not good at absorbing the negative, so tell yourself, "I am not going to fall asleep," and the mind will conversely receive the thought, "I am going to fall asleep." I like to pretend that I am a caregiver that has to stay awake, in order to watch out for a loved one in the next room. Suddenly, because I am denying myself of the chance to sleep, that is all I want to do—sleep. Very shortly thereafter, I am nodding off. Sound crazy? Try it!

Once you are sufficiently sleepy again, with your eyelids closed, roll your eyeballs up. Repeat this several times. When you are actually in a sleep state, your eyeballs randomly roll up, over and over again. By consciously rolling your eyes up, as described, this tricks the mind to bring on the sleep state.

Allow your mind to camp out in your happy place, whatever that is. It can be the beach or the mountains, only you know what your sweet spot looks like. As you do this, surround yourself with a visual experience that engages, at least three of your senses. For example, picture a beautiful, lush green field. Feel the cool, thick carpet of emerald-colored grass beneath your bare feet. As the black clouds are approaching, smell the promise of imminent rain in the air. Enjoy the cool wind while it gently caresses your bare arms, giving you goose bumps. Listen to the trees whisper as they slightly sachet back and forth. Pretty soon you should be relaxed enough to doze off.

More exercises can be found in the E section (http://www.mirror.co.uk/lifestyle/health/unable-sleep-eleven-ways-you-2300449).

Rituals are comforting. So, initially follow a schedule and stick to it religiously, especially if your insomnia is severe. It is very important, when dealing with insomnia, to train your mind to recognize when it's time to slow down. You have to discipline your overactive mind, because so many things compete for its attention. The mind makes associations that produce reactions. For example, if you're a person that walks the dog, drinks a small glass of water, lays out your clothes for the next day, showers, and then turns in for the night, all of those little steps prepare your mind to settle and welcome sleep.

Here's a tried and true schedule you can implement. The following recommendations, from *Consumer Reports,* are based on the results of a recent expert survey (*Consumer Reports,* February 2016, p. 31):

7:00 a.m. It's not the best tactic to sleep in—better to get up, even on the weekends, at the same time every day. Your sleep cycle needs the predictability. Remember, you are training your mind!!!

7:30 a.m. To set a proper 24-hour clock, come in contact with the sunshine as soon as possible. This is easy for me because I have to take the dogs out first thing. Open the curtains. Expose yourself to sunlight.

8:00 a.m. If you can squeeze in at least 20 minutes of exercise in the morning, that is great. Regular exercise, as we have discussed and will further explore, aids you in promoting sounder sleep. Go on a brisk walk or ride a stationary bike. For the majority of people, it is better to exercise in the morning than the evening. Most people, you may be different, need to avoid exercise an hour or two before bed.

10:00 a.m. For coffee lovers, you need to have your last cup no later than ten in the morning. Avoid caffeine for at least 6 hours before bed. It's best if you can cut it out, altogether—especially if you have exhausted your adrenal glands. If you suffer from severe insomnia, your adrenals need to be babied. Caffeine stresses the adrenals.

Noon. More sunlight is called for if you want to strengthen your 24-hour sleep cycle. Make sure to take a break and go outside, if you can—even if you have windows.

3:00 p.m. This one is tough for me and on rare occasions, I don't follow my own advice. I love naps, as I have already covered in previous material. But the experts all say, for chronic insomnia, skip the naps. You can take a nap if you lose some Zzz's one night here or there, but if you have ongoing sleep issues, force yourself to stay awake and give sleep every chance to return the next evening.

6:00 p.m. Early dinners are best for sleep. I guess you're learning; I am the mother of repetition—because repetition is the mother of retention. Avoid big, heavy meals. Sleep is for restoration, not digestion. Have your alcohol several hours before bedtime. Wine will help you conk out but you will arouse in the middle of the night and possibly be unable to get back to sleep. Alcohol causes you to wake up earlier than you need to. Bottom line, you lose sleep when you drink too heavily and too close to bedtime.

Now We Are Truly Entering the Quiet Zone
9:00 p.m. Power down electrical devices just like you would on a plane when preparing for landing. The lights from these gadgets and the TV hamper the release of melatonin, your sleep hormone. So much has already been said about this that your head is probably spinning. I wish I could reach out to you and snatch all the gadgets right out of your hand—ev-

ery night at 9 p.m. on the dot. The TV should be turned off, as well. (There is an 80/20 rule of grace that I reviewed with you in the overview section of Restorative Sleep. But for more severe cases of insomnia, you need to be as militant as you can in your efforts to stick to a schedule.)

10:00 p.m. This is where the real fun begins and your mind is being disciplined—by setting the stage for sleep. You want to give sleep the royal treatment and roll out the red carpet, figuratively—not literally. Unfortunately, red is a very energetic color and is typically not used in a bedroom. So roll out a sleep carpet that is a muted color. This is a wonderful hour where you power down your brain. Dim the bedroom lights— have the softest reading light bulbs for the bedroom. Read a book with real pages that you can touch and turn—no electrical gadgets. Light a candle (remember to put it out before dozing off), drink warm milk (more on this in the N chapter for nutrition). Play quiet, relaxing music, meditate, look at magazines that relax you, and write thank you notes or journal. Just enjoy this time in your bed soaking up the beauty of retreat. Avoid all TV at this point. DVR shows you don't want to miss.

10:55 p.m. Sensory deprivation measures must be deployed at this point like clockwork. Close the curtains or pull down the shades; darken the room as best you can. Make sure all those pesky tiny colored lights—red, green, blue, white, or yellow, whatever they may be, from various electrical devices—are covered with tape. Put your eyeshades on, insert your earplugs, or turn on your white noise of choice; perhaps it is a phone app or a real fan or possibly a sound machine. You need to be "full on" in your battle against insomnia. This is war. But at the same time, you need to be completely relaxed.

11:00 p.m. Whatever you do, try to go timeless. Do not watch the clock. Watching the minutes go by can cause you to panic, which is never good for drifting off to sleep. Place your phone under the bed while it charges and turn it off. If you do look at your clock, there are sleep apps that keep the screen of your iPhone from being disruptive to your melatonin.

3:00 a.m. Waking up at 3:00 a.m. can be a sign of depression. So make note of that and deal with it in more depth with the appropriate professional clinician if this becomes chronic. But when you wake up at 3 a.m. and can't go back to sleep after 20 minutes, you may want to get up and go in another room. Do something relaxing. If you read, it needs to be from a conventional book and not a handheld device.

The remaining sections—sections R, S, and E—also touch on the subject of uncluttering the mind for sound sleep. The E section (E for Exercise) addresses mental and deep breathing exercises for clearing the mind. The S section helps unclutter the mind by focusing on the more spiritual approach to sleep—through the renewing of your mind with Scripture.

The next section—R of the N.U.R.S.E. acronym, is dedicated to the question, "What's keeping you up at night?" Thoughts, concerning all sorts of lifestyle issues, such as your relationships, particularly the toxic ones, can cause your mind to race at night. But I saved the bedroom partner—your most important earthly relationship, for this section—U: uncluttering the heart for better sleep.

UNCLUTTERING YOUR HEART FOR SLEEP

Your spouse, your sweetheart, your bedroom partner, should be your very best friend. Together, you both should be the safest place for each other on planet earth. Keep watch over each other's heart with love and respect. Even when you are at odds, always be kind. If you are out in the world every day, you know how the world beats each of you up on a daily basis. This special person you've chosen to share your life with deserves your kindest voice and most respectful words. Don't allow unresolved anger into your sleep reverie. Guard the benediction to your day and protect yourself from anything that robs you of peace—and ultimately, sleep.

The one you choose to be your partner, in life and love, should be a careful, thoughtful, as well as, a prayerful choice. If this prospect is problematic before you marry, they will be worse after they no longer have to be on their best behavior to snag you. If they are unnecessarily rude and over the top, with outbursts of anger while you are in the dating stage, it will only get worse after the "I do's."

There is this thought out there, and I agree—Go into marriage with your eyes wide open, and once married keep them half shut. Look for patterns and when someone tells you who they are—believe them, but especially when someone shows you who they are—believe them! Even in the simple, nontoxic declarations, if someone says, "I don't like to stay up late." Believe them and respect who they are; don't try to change them.

No matter what the stage is, of a relationship or marriage— even if you live in separate cities, you need to resolve the conflict by phone (texting is a cop out). And again, never go to bed with unresolved anger. Agree to disagree, but at least be kind to one another, honoring each other with the words you choose. Starting the day with left over anger from the night before is poison to the fresh, new 24 hours—so full of promise.

> *"Be angry, and yet do not sin;*
> *do not let the sun go down on your anger"*
> (Ephesians 4:26).

In serious, heated debates, be the bigger person and say something like, "I know we don't see eye to eye on this, but I want to be fair, so I am going to get some sleep and pick this up when I am rested. I love you and want us to resolve this as soon as we can. I am committed to trying to understand your point of view, and I would ask you to do the same."

If you are physically near one another, at the very least, give each other a heart-felt hug before turning in for the night. Emotions may still be raging, depending on the issue, but hopefully, they will have dissipated enough for sleep to overtake you.

You should turn in at the same time as your partner. This builds intimacy—but if one or the other of you, can't fall asleep and wants to leave the room to read or watch TV, at least see your partner off to sleep before you leave the room. If at all possible, both of you should try to be on the same timetable when retiring and rising. This may require some concessions and a bit of working together, to discover a harmonious sleep schedule—but it is well worth the effort.

This bears repeating from the overview section. Research suggests that couples practicing sex are more orgasmic when both participants are properly prepared for a good night's sleep. The release of wonderful hormones produces an "oxytocin" effect, facilitating a more balanced ensemble of cortisol and sex hormones—the perfect setup for mutually sounder sleep to ensue.

When Amanda, our fictitious character from *Holiday*, first saw Graham at her front door, there was an instant attraction and within minutes, she was in bed with him. They were like bunnies from that moment on, enjoying great sex. It worked for them. But that is the typical Hollywood storyline—ever so, nonchalantly, weaving into the script, that the only indicator needed to determine if you're "a match made in heaven"—is the quality of the sex. What a lie! And so many lives have been ruined because they bought the lie. Have you bought the lie?

While a robust sex life is a good thing—you don't just jump in bed with someone within the first ten minutes of meeting them—and end up with a happily-ever-after story.

You may wonder, "Why in the world would you address this matter in a book about sleep?"

Even though, I may lose a good portion of my readers, I so care about each one of you—especially our sons (yes, our sons) and daughters—it's worth the risk I'm taking. The bedroom is for sleep and intimacy, and I want young people to have a fighting chance at enjoying this vital part of their future. This generation is under attack, in these two areas of sleep and intimacy. So I want to give you, or someone you know and love, some needed guidance.

Sex bonds you to the other person, whether you are compatible or not. And if it doesn't, perhaps you've become unable to bond. Like a piece of tape that no longer sticks to anything, because it's adhered to too many objects, over and over again—you can truly lose your ability to bond. Fortunately, there is hope. You can learn how to recover this lost aspect of your personhood. However, it takes a lot of prayer, healing, and time to restore this part of your soul.

Since we are discussing the bedroom, which again, was designed for sleep and intimacy, you may want to revisit some very powerful truths. Truths that today's culture has abandoned—with little to no interest in ever honoring again. This is known as progressive thinking.

Progressives are masters at labeling an idea, referring to it as the very opposite of what it actually is. When something is precious, but is treated in a cavalier manner, i.e., your virginity or chastity—you know what happens? It loses its value. I call that regressive not progressive.

Value your sexuality and who you are. Don't be so eager to give yourself away. Ask yourself, "If I had a house on the market that I wanted to sell, would I allow someone to come and live in my house for free, just to try it out?" They would need to buy it before they moved in, and it's not for rent—it is only for sale. So, no renting either. The interested party needs to show up with all the funds due at closing and buy the house before moving in. Apply the same logic to your dating life. My dear, if he can't afford to marry you, he can't afford you. And for your own good, there should be no permanent, physical bonding through sex until he's equipped to provide for and marry you.

I want to illustrate something to you that no one seems to be talking about by reverting to the previous analogy of tape and bonding through physical intimacy. Because I am making a fleshy example, I'm going to use the example of flesh colored tape—which I buy when I can find it, to cover up cuts or scratches until they heal, especially bug bites to avoid scarring. If you take this tape, or any other type tape for that matter, and you put the two sticky sides together, you will obviously find that it is next to impossible to separate the two pieces of tape without tearing either of the pieces.

Even if you are able to separate the two without tearing them, in any way—good luck with that—eventually, the pieces of tape will start to lose the ability to stick.

Try taking a piece of regular scotch tape and sticking it to a painted wall. Once you carefully remove it, look at the paint residue on the sticky part of the tape. This illustrates how that sticky side of the tape, once applied, is never the same. It will still stick again but not as cohesively. The more the tape is used, the less likely it will effectively stick in the future.

God designed you so that when you have sex, it is a bonding (sticking) to the person and it is meant to last—like the two pieces of tape stuck together. God's idea for sex was marriage, with one person. He wanted that bond to be sealed through the act of sex. Just like the clear piece of tape from the wall, with paint residue on the sticky side. Once it's removed, you will have residue when you are physically intimate—and that was God's intention. He wanted you to become one with your partner, so part of that person will forever be with you and you with them.

Another consideration is all the venereal diseases. You should go online and look at a herpes blister. It looks exactly like someone put tape on your genitalia, consequentially, pulling off tender flesh while removing the tape.

If you are the typical teenager that starts having sex, you are setting yourself up for some real disappointment. You haven't even fully become who you are going to be, and most likely, you are not ready to bond to another at this young age. Therefore, it is not wise to engage in sex. Obviously, teen sex presents the highest probability for getting hurt, because the chances of bonding are so great the first few times.

You will be like the two pieces of flesh tape that tears apart—due to the bond that was formed. But as time marches on, you will learn to adapt and become more casual—more calloused—when it comes to sexual activity, because, just like scar tissue forms after a wound, the tissue is altered, which is a picture of what happens to your soul—your personality. Like scar tissue, you will harden and not be as tender, vulnerable, or trusting. You will be guarded more than you need to be. You don't necessarily have to be aware of it for this to happen.

Beyond the physical consequences, those of you who take the sex act lightly or casually, will lose pieces of yourself. Ultimately, you will be unable to bond in the way God meant for you to bond with your life partner. God's standards are higher, because He wants you to experience the best that life has to offer. If you don't do it His way, you'll never know how good it can be when you do it His way. Somebody out there is waiting for you—hoping you get this right. They deserve the best, so make sure you qualify to be the best.

It's amazing to me that the millennials (and you may be one) are taught to be supersensitive and easily offended. The new term for these misguided souls is "snowflakes." They now believe they are privy to safe places at the schools and on college campuses—just because someone has an opposing thought to theirs. It doesn't matter how small the opposition, they see it as an offense. We need to love them while we toughen them up—for their own good and the overall good of society!

You know this supersensitive mentality will not prevail once these millennials try to make it in the "real" world. You need thick skin to survive in this "dog eat dog" world. Ironically, the call for sensitivity, in true matters of the heart, especially regarding sexual intimacy—often ridiculed by the very schools that espouse the importance of tip-toeing around everyone's thin skin—is nowhere to be found.

Many college campuses promote that students should oblige every sexual whim—no matter how offensive. They tell you not to worry about who or what is in the restroom with you; to be cavalier and recreational when it comes to sex. Basically, they tell you to "deal with it," no matter what the perversion or offense. Tragically, the belief that our youth can and should participate in recreational sex is fairly consistent with what the world believes and teaches. This low standard for our precious young people is considered to be mainstream—before and beyond the college campus. Therefore, you probably won't hear the following ideas from many others.

There is an enemy of your soul. He owns the media, the education system, entertainment, and the cosmos. He is the prince of this world. But the King of kings and Lord of lords is the ultimate Truth. Your Creator knows you intimately—He made you and wants you to have abundant life. The prince of this world is diametrically opposed to God's good plans for you. The enemy of your soul wants to bring death to your future hopes and dreams. I am giving you this truth because few will tell you what the truth really is—in our "politically correct" world!

"The thief comes to steal, kill, and destroy;
I came that they might have life
and have it more abundantly."
(John 10:10).

"For as the heavens are higher than the earth,
So are My ways higher than your ways
And My thoughts than your thoughts"
(Isaiah 55:9).

You acquire soul ties that you were never intended to have through casual sex. What does that mean? Soul ties are emotional, willful, and mindful attachments from previous relationships that you carry with you wherever you go. You may no longer be with a certain person, but soul ties from that person will continue to influence you, having too much subconscious sway over your thoughts and decision making.

Perhaps you are learning about and enjoying a new person, but you will be dealing with old patterns of thinking from the previous relationships—and at a much deeper level, if you were sexually active in any of those partnerships. This is where bonding gets more difficult, the more you give yourself away, the more residual from the previous relationships you will carry with you into future relationships.

This is not just for teens. Recently, I learned of a regrettable situation, where a woman failed to guard her heart. As a result, she was unable to sleep for months—in part, because of debilitating anxiety due to this very matter. To her, sex was recreational—like baseball. In her mind, it was okay to engage in sex with one man after the next, until she was about to be married.

Sporting a carefree facade in this area of her life—as though she had somehow gotten around this truth—she was completely fragile when she finally realized the consequences.

She did not know to what degree her heart was attached to this recreational sex—or this "I'm getting to know you" sex. Buying the Hollywood lie, she ended up with some serious emotional issues. Once it all caught up with her, she received treatment and counsel for her anxiety and debilitating insomnia. Thankfully, she went on to discover complete restoration and overcame her crippling insomnia. Just like the woman at the well (John 4:7-27), Jesus met her with Grace and delivered her from serial broken relationships when she found true love.

God created sex. It is very much like fire, however. Both sex and fire are beautiful, warm, and purposeful in the right context—yet, devastating and destructive in the wrong context. Fire in the fireplace is beautiful, but fire on the couch is a disaster! Sex outside of marriage will hurt you. Maybe immediately—or maybe not—but eventually, you will suffer the consequences. You may not ever realize how it has hurt you, especially since you won't know what you could have enjoyed if you had waited and followed God's principles.

Once, someone wisely said that there is no condom for the heart. Ladies, you have the most to gain by waiting and doing it God's way and the most to lose by ignoring God's will for you. As a nurse, I can tell you, your very anatomy works against you, because your sexual organs are internal, and the guy's sexual organs are external. The sex act affects you to a greater degree psychologically and emotionally. This is by God's design. He created men to be tougher—to be the protectors—and women to be more tender; the nurturers.

The consequences for sex outside of marriage are greater by far for women. You will sleep much better—when you finally find your life partner—if you don't bring memories of other partners or diseases to the bed. Incidentally, I haven't even touched on unwanted pregnancies and abortions. Nor have I mentioned the growing problem of pornography among our young men and even boys. Several mothers have confessed this is a great concern for our sons. This ultimately, comes back to young girls being seen as objects to be used, rather than precious souls to be cherished.

Sadly, I am being told that currently most of the teenagers are having sex. So parents, you are allowing them to take the pill, based on your own very real fears. However, I believe, if you talk to them and teach them these truths—early enough and all along the way—they can reach for, and enjoy, higher standards. Give them a chance, by helping them understand these consequences and empowering them to make right choices. They may surprise you and opt for a better life—but not if they never hear the truth from you.

I realize the ideal doesn't always happen. So, you need to know, you can get your chastity back—not your virginity, but your chastity. Now, there's a word you never hear anymore.

Jon Weece, author of *Me Too: Experience the God Who Understands*, points out the way to build community and find like-minded people is to start with the words, "Me, too." You and I live in a fallen world, and we are all striving to be the best we can be. So, reach out and find people who share your values.

The Bible refers to this concept as being "equally yoked." Jesus showed us His human side with His struggles in the Garden of Gethsemane. This was one of His greatest "Me, too" moments. He is fully acquainted with you and your struggles, meeting you at your most vulnerable point, helping you make the best decisions. Trust Him. If you do, He will lead you to the right people. (There is more about this in the next R section.)

I also suggest you read, *And the Bride Wore White*, by Dannah Gresh.

"Therefore, there is now no condemnation

for those who are in Christ Jesus"
(Romans 8:1).

Let your bedroom be all God intended for it to be and enjoy the intimate side of sleep.

Remember, He works the night shift, so you don't have to do anything but sleep. Give Him your cares, and He will provide the rest you need.

Here's a prayer that might be meaningful for you to pray:

Father,
Help me take back the part of me that I gave to others,
by being intimate, when this was not Your choice for me.
Help me give back the parts I took from others, as well.
I thank You, Lord, that You are untying the soul strings,
that I have been living with—causing me to live like a
puppet in bondage to others. I surrender to You my
soul ties and exchange them for Your peace and
abundant living. You are setting me free and giving me sweet
sleep. Thank You for Your love, tender mercies and forgiveness.
I rest in Your grace. My heart is at peace by faith. Help me
follow Your will for my life and be obedient to Your ways.
In Your Name.

SLEEP Q-TIPS:

- If you read at night, read from a book—not from a handheld device.

- Make the room as pitch dark as possible. Place tape over scattered artificial lights, such as, red buttons on devices or glowing clocks. Or wear a sleep mask to cover your eyes. (Moonlight doesn't destroy melatonin as readily.)

- No mirrors in the bedroom. It's even better if there is no TV.

- Buy the best pillows and mattress you can afford.
- Your mattress should be replaced every eight years, if used regularly.
- Flip and rotate your mattress every season; Winter, Spring, Summer, and Fall.
- Buy new pillows once they get lumpy.
- Use the highest quality cotton sheets you can afford.
- Clean sheets are best for sleep, so have enough sets to wash and rotate often.
- Take a relaxing shower or hot bath prior to retiring.
- You may want to add some valerian root to your bath water for some relaxation in preparation for sleep. It is reported to work wonders for insomnia.
- For winter months, have a top sheet, then a blanket, or a thin quilt—a matelassé—in summer months. On top of the blanket, have another top sheet all tucked in. This allows for more comfortable sleep.
- Use your iPhone flashlight or a small flashlight for night trips to the restroom to keep you from turning on too much light, affecting your melatonin. I have seen plug-in and leave-in night lights that operate as motion sensors. They light up softly when they detect motion. Research conducted by the National Institutes of Health reveals that the slightest light exposure suppresses melatonin production in lab animals: a one minute exposure to white light every two hours during the night suppressed melatonin production by 65%. Red light however, is the only type of light that does not affect melatonin production. Try this product: (Pack of 2) Iavo Auto ON/OFF Plug In LED Night Light with Dusk to Dawn Sensor (Pink/Red).
- Lavender scents, packaged in a variety of forms, such as

candles, can promote sleep—but must be put out before the final doze.

- Wash your pajamas in a lavender-scented softener.

- Rub a small amount of lavender oil on the ball of your feet.

- Dab some eucalyptus oil on your pillow, if you have trouble breathing, like when you suffer from a cold.

- Invest in a machine that plays white noise to block out sounds from loud people and other noises, or download free apps for your iPhone.

- We have talked about powering down and the adverse effect of hand-held devices which destroys melatonin. However, there are some wonderful new sleep apps designed to help you sleep and monitor your sleep habits. I am not for, or against, them. Check out what's available and decide for yourself (www.healthline.com/health/healthy-sleep/top-in-somnia-iphone-android-apps#3).

- Keep your feet warm, if they are prone to getting cold. Microwavable slippers are excellent for warming your feet, due to poor circulation—but avoid electric blankets.

- Sleeping on your side in the fetal position, or even worse, on your stomach, may be your favorite sleep position, but after years of this habit, your facial collagen will break down, and you will develop wrinkles. Train yourself to sleep on your back, even if you have to buy two body pillows and sleep between them.

- Purchase silk pillowcases. Chinese women have used these for years to curtail the problem of facial wrinkling.

- Change your pillow cases every three days, at the least, to avoid breakouts.

- If you sleep in the fetal position, keep it loose rather than tight, with the chin not buried in your chest. Have a pillow between your knees. The fetal position is best for pregnant women, due to circulation matters related to the baby. According to the National Sleep Foundation, the number one best position is on your back.

- Listen to Scripture lullabies such as, www.scripturelullabies. com, or Scripture being read on www.biblegateway.com (my personal favorites). Choose an apparatus for listening that doesn't glow in the dark, or cover it with a towel or pillow. The artists of these Scripture songs and narrators of Scripture readings are gifted at striking the right tone for nightly listening. The Scriptures will calm anxieties and promote sleep.

- The Latinos, as a culture, know the importance of making your bedroom a success for sleep and intimacy. Latino women are known for their bedroom savvy and wisdom by keeping bedrooms cozy and intimate: They keep the main thing, the main thing by streamlining their bedroom for only two activities: sleep and intimacy. From this culture, I learned to keep the bedroom small. It has been believed by this culture that the bigger the bedroom, the higher the divorce rate.

- Holding hands, as you are drifting off to sleep, has a calming effect. Try holding hands with your partner, as you spoon extra close. It can relax you and help you fall asleep more easily.

- You will sleep much better—when you finally find your life partner—if you don't bring memories of other partners or their diseases to the bed.

- This bears repeating—I realize the ideal doesn't always happen. So, you need to know, you can get your chastity back—not your virginity—but your chastity. Let's be vigilant to teach our sons and daughters it is best to wait, but if you have gotten ahead of yourself, there is still hope to receive God's best. Rest, and receive His best. Don't be anxious. All is well. Remember, someone's hoping you get this right. And when you meet them, you're going to be glad you did.

- Visit Alison A. Armstrong's wonderful website: www.queenscode.com! She is a master at understanding men. Alison has revolutionized the way men and women relate to one another. One of her greatest points of focus is the bedroom.

R: THE N.U.R.S.E. APPROACH TO RESTORATIVE SLEEP:

Remodeling Your Life:
The Five Pillars of Rest

Residence, Resources, Roles, Relationships, and Religion

The critique of Amanda, our fictitious character from the movie, Holiday, establishes the idea that the sleep she is missing is as precious and rare these days as gold. When your sleep account is in overdraft, you pay a great price. You need sleep so you can be your best self and live the life you were created to live. Because sleep is so vital to your overall wellbeing, examine your life to find out what's keeping you up at night.

What drove Amanda to totally remodel her life? A break-up with her boyfriend—due to her workaholic tendencies—which ultimately resulted in her battle with insomnia. Because of her desperate need to resolve this problem, Amanda embarked on a winsome journey that led her to a beautiful new life, filled with people who genuinely loved her. She finally took care of her primary food issue. The N section introduces primary food in greater detail.

*When there is genuine love in your life,
you can overcome almost anything.*

Sometimes, maladies such as, insomnia, cause so much discomfort, these deficits turn out to be gifts—forcing you to deal with areas in your life that may have gone awry. These irritants, if dealt with, can help you create precious pearls. The moment this happens, the world really does become your oyster.

As Amanda's world became her own oyster, her demeanor assumed a whole new glow—like that of a lustrous, rare and precious pearl. Insomnia, the obvious irritant in Amanda's world, forced her to undergo a life-style makeover, resulting in a more harmonious life. Once she made the decision to change, she then allowed time to transition her out of a loveless relationship, into a loving and joy filled life—encompassing family, friends, and loads of fun. As she settled into her new lifestyle, she began to sleep again.

When the cause of your own sleep deprivation eludes you, drill down and examine each aspect of your life. Remind yourself of Amanda, and take the challenge to remodel your life so you can sleep.

Think of a doctor's visit for your annual check-up. You answer pages of questions for your comprehensive history and physical. In the same way, in order to find out what's keeping you up at night, you need to consider a host of questions, representative of five areas in your life that might be in need of some remodeling.

Don't worry if you're not fancy free and single like Amanda. Having a family, and making a living to create a loving home, doesn't mean you're stuck. You may have more responsibilities and challenges, but you can still tweak the life you are living and make the needed improvements. But first get honest with yourself, so you can identify any problem(s) potentially causing you to lose vital sleep at night.

The answer to the question of *"What's keeping you up at night?"* may entail: a lack of **resources**, toxic or challenging **relationships**, or various **roles** you play in your daily living. Or, perhaps you need a change of **residence**, due to a noisy neighbor—above, below, adjacent, or next door to you—acting like a terror at night.

Concerning night terror, with the current world stage, you could actually be dealing with an ominous, but very real threat of terror—not to mention constant media coverage, blasting stories of terrorist attacks 24-7/365, along with *wars and rumors of wars*. Perhaps it's the **religion** of these zealots, threatening our very existence that's contributing to your insomnia.

No matter who you are, where you live, or in what stage of life you find yourself, there is a chance you may have issues in one, or all of these categories—the five pillars of rest. It's time to examine the five pillars of rest in your life—(1) residence, (2) roles, (3) resources, (4) relationships, and (5) religion. It could be that as you look at these five areas, you will discover you need to do some remodeling in your life so that you can once again, sleep soundly.

RESIDENCE

For years, I lived in a small one-bedroom condo that was as sound proof as a cardboard box. The man above me was a curmudgeon who cycled. He would hang his bikes from the ceiling like bats. Often he would drop them on the floor, which was my ceiling, as he was trying to take them down. Four in the morning was his time to wake up and hit the trail with his loud, barking dog. Unfortunately, the dog sported a disfiguring canine brain tumor. Even worse, the man was up all night stomping to and from the restroom. He was an alcoholic with no manners at all! Such a great guy.

One night, at 3 a.m., his dog was at my door barking. While I assessed the situation, the barking dog created quite a bit of commotion, causing my dogs to arouse. Once awake, they needed to go outside and pee. His dog, Maggie, seemed okay, but I didn't know if the now even larger brain tumor might cause her to be aggressive, so I hesitated to fully open the door. All of a sudden, I felt something warm and wet at the hem of my robe. My little maltese decided enough of this waiting. With his leg hiked, like a big dog, he got me good.

Ultimately, I had to brave it and take Maggie upstairs to her owner's apartment, even though I was scared of the dog. Having just survived a dog attack that same summer, I didn't want to risk more scars. Apparently, my upstairs neighbor let her out and left his door open without a light on.

Was the curmudgeon grateful that I helped his lost dog return home? No, he had passed out. Once I got him to wake up, he was unbearably rude—spewing out a mouthful of obscenities. Did I mention he was also the President of the Board for the Condominium Association?

Endless stories could be told, but finally, after seven years, I sold my condo at a $12,000 loss—just so I could get some sleep. Regardless of the situation, no matter what, do your best to buy or rent a unit on the top floor.

Unfortunately, as beautiful as my next apartment was, I still had a similar problem. I rented a lovely terrace-level apartment—not in a condo—but in a freestanding home in a gorgeous gated community, overlooking a golf course. Since there was no insulation, and the bedroom was directly under the kitchen, sleep continued to be a challenge for me. The owner must have slept all day because he was in the kitchen off and on throughout the night. Even though the price was right, and the yard was great for my dogs, I still could not get my needed sleep.

I tried for months on end to sleep. There were two fans

running to create white noise, and I used earplugs to siphon sleepy-time music with Scripture reading into my exhausted ears. Still, I could not drown out the noise from the kitchen. Killing any hope of sleep in my bed, I decided to sleep on the couch in the living room. I did this for weeks until I got sciatica. Finally, I moved my bed into the living room in a desperate attempt to sleep in peace. I guess if I had to give up any of the five senses, it would be hearing! No not really, I take that back. I am actually very grateful for my ears— and my superb hearing.

Currently, I live on the second floor of a four-story condominium. For the most part, I can sleep, but there are nights where I have to employ every one of my strategies and tips just to drown out the noise and sleep.

Examine this area of your life by asking yourself the following questions:

- Do I need to move?

- Can I afford to move?

- What other alternatives are there?

- Have I tried white noise, using a fan, iPhone sleep apps and/or earplugs?

- What are my rights?

- Are my nuisance neighbors in violation of their home-owner's agreements?

- Have I checked city ordinances and state noise laws for apartments and condominiums?

- Have I approached the culprits nicely?

- Are they reasonable?

- Is management involved?

- Have I exhausted all of my options?

- Do I have a good exit strategy for improving the situation? (Be careful to avoid jumping out of the frying pan into the fire.)

You may live in the country—next to a neighbor that has a kennel of loud barking dogs—ready for the early morning hunt. Or maybe you live in a city that never sleeps. Either way, in order to get some *shut-eye,* you must learn to shut out the "hustle and bustle" of night-time, as well as other wee morning, nocturnal activities. Otherwise, just so you can get some uninterrupted sleep, you may seriously need a change of residence.

ROLES

Any time you step out of your mold, it is not uncommon to feel uncomfortable. Sometimes, in order to regain balance in your life, you have to consider making minor or major adjustments. Ultimately, you may be required to enact huge changes. Ask yourself the following questions:

- Am I doing too much?
- Am I involved in too many groups?
- Why am I doing _____?
- Are the activities I am engaged in rewarding?
- Why do I feel compelled to attend_____?
- Am I afraid to say, "No?"
- Would I be happier, if I had more "me" time?
- Is this season in my life over?
- Do I need to move on?
- Have I outgrown this?
- Is this really where I need to be?

- Is this the right group for me?
- Do I really fit in, or is there a better fit for me somewhere else?
- Am I afraid to try something new? And if the answer is yes, why?
- What would I be doing, if I didn't have to worry about earning a living?
- What are my gifts?
- What are my talents?
- What do I really want to do with my life?
- What was I born to do?
- What is my calling?
- Who needs me the most?
- What am I most passionate about curing, changing, fixing, defending, helping or improving?
- Answer this question: "I feel God's pleasure when I_____?"

If you lose a job, then you have no choice but to look for another one, unless you are financially able to do otherwise. Consider how blessed you are if you are counted among these fortunate few.

On occasion, you may need to change jobs, or flat out quit a job—even without having another one. This needs to happen when a work situation becomes abusive or toxic. There are so many clichés about closing one door and opening another, but the truth is this: life has a way of working out, if you just keep on keeping on. Look at your situation as an opportunity—not an obstacle or a hurdle to overcome. Never, ever get so overwhelmed that you give up, no matter what.

I have had to resign from two jobs without having another

one and with each situation, I had no slush fund or cushion. God assured me He would take care of me, through the Scriptures and sermons I heard. Within hours, I had another job in both instances.

With each job loss, I had no nursing skills either time—since I had not done any clinical work in years—I truly could not afford to miss a check. In each circumstance, I prayed and really sought the Lord so that I didn't just quit on a whim. But I knew He did not want me to live like I was living. Thankfully, I was able to get rehired in roles that were more conducive to my skill set. Miraculously, my new jobs did not require traditional nursing skills.

One of the best things you can do—when a change is needed, in either your overall life or just your daily grind—is to get a good night's sleep. This will help you stay alert. Alert people think more clearly. They have better insight and generate more creative ideas. Rested people are fresh and more emotionally stable. You can demonstrate more courage and take calculated risks with better clarity when you are rested.

Sleep deprivation is a side effect of a life that needs examining. Find out what is keeping you up at night and commit to resolving it the best way you can. Make every effort to be well rested, even though your challenging time might cause episodes of insomnia.

When life is really hard and you need sleep the most, this is also the time you may be forced to give it up—especially if you are responsible for providing care to a loved one. This can be an extremely challenging paradox to parents who have crying babies throughout the night. Even more trying is being the caregiver to your spouse. Or being an adult child of an aging parent, who keeps you up throughout the night—especially during the work week, while still having to hold down a job. If at all possible, reach out to your church or synagogue for assistance and referral sources. Oftentimes, friends and family will relieve you for a few hours in the evening or during the day, so you can revamp.

Financial resources are a plus in these situations. If you can afford to hire someone, then the challenge is finding someone you can trust. There are all kinds of organizations to assist you in finding the right resources—such as Sixty Plus and A Place for Mom. They can make recommendations regarding caregivers, daycare for adults, and other ancillary agencies. Ask local hospital staff and your physician to help you find resources to assist you in finding caregivers. Call the case management departments of your local hospitals for the most knowledgeable professionals, who can recommend agencies in your area that you may not have thought to call.

The most comprehensive resource I have found, for caregivers dealing with this matter, is the free manual, *Dealing with Dementia: A Caregiver's Guide*, produced by the Rosalynn Carter Institute for Caregiving. The author left no stone unturned. There is a plethora of information regarding how to help your loved one who has dementia. It entails advice on how to help your loved one get some sleep, as well as manage your own stress and sleep deprivation. In dealing with a loved one with dementia, this handbook includes the contact information for every dementia resource you can imagine. The contact information is:

The Rosalynn Carter Institute for Caregiving
800 Georgia Southwestern State University Drive
Americus, GA 31709-4379
www.rosalynncarter.org
(229)-928-1234 phone Fax: (229) 931-2663
RCICaregiving@gsw.edu
http://www.rosalynncarter.org/caregiver_resources/

"There are only four kinds of people in this world:
- *Those who have been caregivers,*
- *Those who currently are caregivers,*
- *Those who will be caregivers, and*
- *Those who will need caregivers."*

—Rosalynn Carter

Honestly, caregivers are some of the most sleep-deprived people among us. They need our love, support, and prayers. Perhaps you are someone who fits the bill. You would never ask for help but you sure would love for someone to relieve you so you could retreat to your bedroom and sleep without having to worry about your loved one. Or perhaps you know someone that needs your assistance and you could provide that relief.

RESOURCES (FINANCES)

Concerning resources, examine your life by asking yourself the following questions:

- Do I really need all the things I think I do?

- How can I cut back on expenses, so that I am not a borrower who becomes a slave to the lender?

- What do I really want? More stuff? More status? More peace? More freedom?

- How can I obtain relief from the mistakes I've made?

- Do I need to remodel my life, and learn to live on less, so that I can get off of the treadmill?

- Am I doing what I truly want with my life, or am I trying to pay for a life that I really don't enjoy?

- Am I faithful in the little things? Or am I unwise and wasteful concerning money and goods—always asking for more?

• Am I addicted to making money?

• When is enough, enough?

Sometimes it's not enough to have a million dollars; why not a two million, a hundred million, or even a billion? That's all well and good to want to make more money, but not at the expense of your health. If you are staying up, night and day, because you are addicted to making money—and you can't find the off button—in the end, you will have a disappointing finish.

James 4:4 reminds us that friendship with the world is enmity with God. As a believer, you must guard against cozying up to the world and all of its charms. God favors purity of heart and a simple life of faith. In *The Best is Yet to Come*, Ann Platz cautions, the grandiose life of glitz, glamour, and glory offers a slew of temptations that may cause you to forget your God. The Lord knows that somewhere within the zone lies the sweet spot.

In Proverbs 30:8 we read, *"Give me enough food to live on, neither too much nor too little. If I'm too full, I might get independent, saying, 'God? Who needs him?' If I'm poor, I might steal and dishonor the name of God"* (The Message). To be self-sustaining, more often than not, causes people to turn from God because they have all they need. But Agur, the author of the Proverb, also knew how destructive poverty was to a man and his family. So in wisdom he came to God, asking to be given what he needed on middle ground, by simply asking for wisdom rather than riches. Very few people can live on the high extreme end of the spectrum without overtaxing their body to get there. Remember, having more than enough, and being able to help others, is an awesome goal, but burning it at both ends for decades could cost you in the long run. Take care of your mind and vital organs; allow them to sleep.

The adrenal rush from hitting the big time can give you a false sense of energy. The pay-off is huge, when the stakes are high—but living on the edge, day after day, takes a toll. What difference will it make, if you have all the money in the world, but you're walking the halls of a locked Alzheimer's unit because you never slept?

Don't buy the lie you may have sold yourself and can't afford to believe—the lie that you don't need as much sleep as everybody else. Maybe you do and maybe you don't, but by the time you find out, it may be too late. You need to ask yourself, "Do I want to be a burden to my family? Am I taking care of myself, so that I'm not at a high risk for developing a devastating disease, such as Alzheimer's, as a direct result of chronic insomnia?"

According to a headline in the *Atlanta Journal-Constitution*, "The Cost of Alzheimer's Can Devastate a Family's Finances." On average, the cost is as follows:

- $21: Hourly rate for home health care.

- $70: Daily rate for adult day care.

- $87,235: Annual rate for a private room in the nursing home. (Medicare does not cover a private room, unless the patient is contagious. And it only pays for the first 100 days; 100% for the first 20 days, and on day 21 it drops to 80%. If there is no secondary policy through commercial insurance or Medicaid, the patient has to pay out of pocket for the copayment. The average length of stay is between 800–900 days for the entire duration of the Alzheimer's care.)

- $174,000: Average lifetime cost of care for an Alzheimer's patient.

- $33.6 billion: Annual loss of productivity to the overall

national economy by family care givers—leaving the work force to care for Alzheimer's patients.

- $183 billion: Overall cost for Alzheimer's patients in 2011.
- $1.1 trillion: Projected overall cost for Alzheimer's patients in 2050.

These are some facts, according to the Alzheimer's Association, related to caregivers for family members suffering with Alzheimer's:

- Two thirds of caregivers are women, and 34% of these women are over 65, resulting in an estimated 17.9 billion hours of unpaid care.

- Forty-one percent of the caregivers have an income of $50K/year.

- These caregivers are emotionally exhausted; about 40% understandably report suffering from depression.

Ann Platz, previously referred to, has written a charming book, *The Best Is Yet to Come*. It proclaims that life is all about progressing from one season to the next. If you are living a disciplined life, with God at the center, naturally, the best season of all should be the next one ahead. As you progress through life and grow in your walk with the Lord, the ultimate goal is always to increase your intimacy with Him. Without steadily growing in intimacy with Jesus, you don't know what you are missing. I am reminded of the old song, *The Longer I Serve Him, the Sweeter He Grows*. The title says it all. Sadly, Alzheimer's is a huge threat to the hope that the best is yet to come.

Take care of yourself. Do whatever it takes to get the adequate sleep you need, so that your loved ones are not burdened with this devastating disease. This was covered in part one, but sleep deprivation is believed to be a major contributing factor to dementia and Alzheimer's.

Workaholics, burning it at both ends—like Amanda, our fictitious character—suffer from devastating consequences of ignoring their personal lives, one of which is chronic insomnia. The other side of the insomnia coin is a lack of resources. Unemployment can banish any hope of sleep. The unemployment rate is staggering right now. Even though it may get better or worse, it boils down to possessing the ability to earn your own living. Having a livelihood, which empowers you to make a decent life for yourself, is mandatory to living an optimal life. Is it time to get current with more hirable skills, while you're also getting current on your Zzz's?

"But if anyone does not provide for his own,
and especially for those of his household, he has denied
the faith and is worse than an unbeliever"
(1 Timothy 5:8).

The bottom line is to do everything in moderation—including moderation. Sometimes you have to turn it up a notch. You may have to bust it for a season, but know your limits and listen to your body. Working two jobs for a season is doable, but always take care of yourself. Live within your means and don't presume on the future. Be a good partner and provider for your household by making wise decisions. Implement some third stage thinking and ask yourself, "Is this what I need to do in order to reap a good harvest in the long run?"

Take care of your body so you can finish well. There are circumstances that call for an all-out, over-the-top push to get ahead. But this has to be for a season—not a way of living. Chasing money is foolish. Chasing God is wise.

Learn to make the most of whatever season you are in. Set goals that stretch you so the next season becomes progressively better. Again, moderation is the key. Always incorporate restorative sleep into your planning, so you can enjoy the harvest when it finally comes.

Be grateful for the season you are in, and enjoy life to the fullest—while you continue to strive to be your best. Always live with an attitude of gratitude. If you are having trouble sleeping, because you are worried, think of the movie, *It's a Wonderful Life*.

Imagine what life would be like if you only woke up to the things you remembered to thank God for—the night before. Isn't that what Clarence, the angel, taught George (Jimmy Stewart) in *It's a Wonderful Life?* Clarence showed George what the world would be like if he had never been born? Because of crippling debt, George questioned whether his life had any value? Just as he was about to jump off a bridge, his angel came to the rescue. Due to the angelic ability of Clarence—to reveal the back story of all the events of George's life—George finally recognizes his life really is full of reasons to truly celebrate.

When you are buried in debt and feel so overwhelmed that you can't sleep at night, a great place to start is Dave Ramsey's, *Financial Peace University*—a course for getting out of debt. It also teaches you how to live debt-free. Dave is famous for saying that a paid off mortgage is the new status symbol of choice—replacing the BMW.

Most synagogues and churches offer free assistance and similar tools to help you manage finances and get you out of debt— in the shortest amount of time. Your local library is another resource for finding helpful information.

Getting support and having accountability helps you stay motivated, to make course corrections in your finances and avoid feeling all alone. There is a principle to which I ascribe. It is an oxymoron to some, but God has an upside down economy. *"Give and it shall be given unto you"* (Luke 6:38 KJV). This is what the Scriptures teach. Give your way out of debt.

No matter how broke you may be, you can give something. Giving unclogs the flow of blessing.

When I was in college, I was a summer camp counselor for young girls. This was a little song we sang when we gave our offerings:

"Giving is not subtracting,
It's adding, don't you see?
What you lose becomes another's gain.
Sharing is not dividing,
It's multiplying life.
Like the flowers after morning rain."

Don't you love God's math? God supplies all of our needs, according to His riches in glory. He does not want anyone to lose sleep over a lack of resources. (We will look at this in more detail is the S chapter of the N.U.R.S.E. Approach to Restorative Sleep.)

RELATIONSHIPS

Be wise as a serpent and harmless as a dove, when it comes to relationships. In other words, be gentle with people. Give them the benefit of the doubt and extend grace to everyone— but don't be foolish. When forming friendships, you should operate like a convertible—learn to put the top up when you see a storm brewing. Otherwise, you might get drenched. Set boundaries, keep them, and you'll sleep much sounder.

Regarding the people you have in your life, ask **yourself** the following questions to determine what might be keeping you up at night:

- Do the people in my life bring out the best in me?
- Do I like who I am, when I am around them?
- Can I truly be my authentic self?

- Are those around me easy to be with?
- Do they cause static in my life? Or, do they cause peace to reign?
- Are they fun?
- Do they major on the minors?
- Are they petty?
- Are they whisperers?
- Do they make me laugh?
- Do they make my life better? If yes, how? If not, why?
- Are they full of drama?
- Are they forgiving?
- Do they teach me new and interesting things?
- Do they cause me to grow?
- Do they make me glow? (not from sweat but from their radiant joy!)
- Do they listen to me, or are they always waiting to tell me their woes?
- Are they high maintenance?
- Are they always causing me to have chatter in my head after they leave? (Do I always wish I could clarify one more thing with them?)
- Are they always taking and never giving?
- Do they "get" me?
- Do they celebrate me or just tolerate me?
- Do they offer me constructive criticism versus putting me down?
- Do they genuinely want the best for me, or are they con-

niving and manipulative?

- Are they always competing to "one up" me?
- Are they "okay" with embarrassing or shaming me?
- Are they punitive?
- Are they wise?
- Do I respect them? Do they respect me? If not, why?
- Do I miss them when they are not around, or am I glad to see them go?
- Do I trust them? Do they trust me? If not, why?
- Do they challenge me in a good way?
- Are they always second-guessing me?
- Are they interested in conflict resolution? Or do they just like a good fight?
- Do they want more from me than I can or am willing to give?
- Have I been honest with them?
- Do I want more from them than they can or are willing to give?
- Have they been honest with me?
- Have I been honest with myself about them?
- Have I asked God to show me my blind spots?
- Have I offended them in any way—even if I don't think they are justified?
- Do I need to apologize?
- Have they disrespected me unjustly? If yes, why am I allowing it to continue?
- Do they think they are better than me?

- Am I being disciplined by God through this person?
- Do they have an unjust—morally, superior attitude?
- What new truth do I need to learn?
- Are they my peer? If not, do they think they are?
- Are they overstepping their boundaries?
- Are they controlling?
- Are they unjustly judgmental?

Don't just blow through these questions. Ask the Lord to help you really get still and examine your heart against the backdrop of this list. Go over the list several times and prayerfully answer these questions.

If you don't like the answers to any of these questions, perhaps you have a toxic person or toxic people in your life. When you purge your private life of toxic people, or learn to set and enforce boundaries with all people, your sleep problems will drastically improve.

What does setting boundaries look like? Well, imagine your life is a stage, and there is a huge stage curtain—also known as a grand drape, act curtain, house curtain, house drape or main drape. The players on the stage, acting out the scenes with you, represent the people in the inner most circle of your life—usually loved ones and family members.

Then there are front row friends that are able to see your life up close. These are people that you should trust, people to whom you have earned their respect.

Toxic people are balcony people. They should be kept at bay. The really toxic people, such as coworkers in your life with whom you have to associate—but not by choice, are lobby people.

Love is the curtain rod that the grand drape hangs on. You determine who is in your inner circle and who has a front row seat to your life, but the curtain always opens and closes on the rod of love. Walk the line of "love" with all people, but also set boundaries. God loves toxic people. He also loves you so lavishly that you can afford to love these misfortunate souls— no matter how challenging their behavior may be.

Toxic People Will Keep You Up at Night

I can make the case that all toxic behavior is rooted in fear. You are either a person of faith or you are a person of fear. Faith is your friend and fear is your enemy. In life, faith brings you what you want; fear brings you what you don't want. Faith and fear work the same way. Both bring you what you focus on and confess.

However, fear is the worst form of bondage. It robs you and those around you of seeing your goals and dreams thrive. Ultimately, for the purpose of this subject, fear robs you of precious sleep. Perhaps you need to send your own "pet fears" out the door and watch insomnia exit with them.

Fear knocks at your door every day, and it will continue to do so as long as you live. If you expose yourself to any kind of news through the Internet, radio, television, or news journals—if you have a conversation with another human being— you have the opportunity to align yourself with fear. Keep fear locked out and tell it to go far away.

Think about it. No one wants to be labeled a fearful person. You hear of millions across the country attending *Women of Faith* conferences. How many people would attend if it were a *Women of Fear* conference? You have a life to live. Make it a well-rested, and faith-filled life. You only get one go at life; there are no do-overs. So, refuse to allow fear to reign in your life. Give fear no place in your life. Since the Bible is our offensive weapon against fear, replace all fearful thoughts with truths from Scripture. Faith comes by hearing the Word of God. Live by faith and sleep in perfect peace.

2 Timothy 1:7 tells us, *"God did not give us a spirit of fear but of love, power and a sound mind."* Fear undermines you and steals your confidence. It causes your mind to race at night, rehearsing all kinds of undesirable scenarios. You awaken to a new day exhausted and short-changed, because you did not fully rest. Let go and allow God to handle the various details of your life, while you retire to dreamland. This will empower you to face the next day with more vigor and resolve. (More on this in the next section: The Spiritual Side of Sleep.)

Frenemies

Look out for the really toxic people that wreak havoc in your life. Take, for example a *"frenemy"*—someone who you would normally like and vice versa. But because of competing agendas and their growing dislike or jealousy of you, they continually undermine you.

Frenemies like you, as long as you never outshine them—and they make it their business to see that you never do. Beware of them. Some people are really crafty, and they can easily fool you. They will try to sabotage your overall success in any given area of your life. *Frenemies* are driven by the fear that you will matter more than they do. These fragile people are excellent at keeping you tossing and turning throughout the night.

Often, a *frenemy* shows up in the workplace, but they can be found almost anywhere—even in your inner circle. You've heard people say, "Keep your friends close and your enemies closer." The idea is to keep a careful eye on those who are out to get you. God ultimately has your back so there is no need to be paranoid. Just be wise to their ways.

If you realize there is a *frenemy* in your inner circle, pray for them, but start to distance yourself by being very discreet regarding the amount of time you spend with them. Guard your words, and be careful what you tell them. To be wise, you probably shouldn't "break bread" with them—not if a good night's sleep is your goal.

Just remember there are countless examples of *frenemies* in the Bible. God uses *frenemies* to promote His people. Think of King Saul and David. God used Saul's jealousy to work in David's life—to produce godly character qualities necessary to be king. While Saul wore the crown, he pursued David for ten years, with the intent to kill him. David was in hiding, on the run from Saul for an entire decade.

Also, our Lord had to deal with Judas. But even as he was betraying Jesus, Judas helped the Son of God fulfill His Father's perfect will.

Lying in bed, while trying to sleep through salty tears—because one of your dearest friends has slowly but surely revealed herself to be a *frenemy*—is the perfect recipe for insomnia. When she ices you out of her life and tries to take a few dear friends with her, the best thing to do is thank God for the wonderful years of friendship you had together. Pray that God blesses her in a way that is meaningful. In your heart, forgive her and thank her for helping you become stronger. Then, move on, free from the sting of her malice.

Thank God for her rejection because it is shaping you into His image. He tells you to pray for those who despitefully use you. When you experience this type of pain, you become more sensitive to the needs of others. You become more compassionate. You grow and mature, even though you would never sign up for this kind of suffering voluntarily.

When you realize that all rejection is God's protection, it takes the sting out of the offense. You can know that for all the times you were there for your friend—even though he or she is not there for you in your hour of need—God will provide the right people to see you through. This is good news for the insomniac.

God gave His life for you, and He loves you with a fierce love. He will never forsake you. Enjoy His lavish love, if you are in a season of abandonment or betrayal. Let Him cover you with His sweet presence and sleep in peace. In the end, people who turn out to be *frenemies* are driven by deep insecurities and fears. These limitations often cause them to be very controlling—either subtly or obtusely—and they are very effective at it.

Frenemies are also very persuasive at aligning others with their way of thinking, causing even close friends to turn away from you. This can be very hurtful but again, pray for them and rest in knowing the Lord has your back. He will see you through and deal with your *frenemy* accordingly.

Let me caution you, though. When the Lord does start spanking your *frenemy*, don't get cocky and start rejoicing, or He may stop disciplining them. Pray for them because, in the end, your *frenemy* may come crawling to you for the help they desperately need.

Henny Pennies

Fearful people—people who live with fear as the backdrop of everything they say and do—are exhausting and will eventually cause disarray in your life. They are always looking for the "sky to fall." When their dire predictions finally manifest, they are actually relieved, because it validates their existence, empowering them to rally the troops. These people are whisperers. They say things like:

"Did I not say that was going to happen?"

"What is she thinking?"

"I can't believe she did that!"

"You can't go there. It's too dangerous."

"You'll never be able to afford that."

"He hasn't suffered enough."

"He needs lots of pain in his life before he will change."

(These people don't realize the Bible teaches—*the kindness of God causes men to repent*.)

It's amazing how much better life is, and how sweet sleep becomes, when you rid your life of the fearful rhetoric of Henny Pennies. I have so much grace for a variety of people and their various challenges, but fearful Henny Pennies seem to run right up on my Achilles heel—more than any other individuals I know. It's as if they are always screaming, "fire," while you're trying to watch the movie, but the only fire to be found is on the panoramic screen. They steal "the moment," just like they steal the "joy" out of life.

I saw this on Facebook once and loved it: *People who want to believe the worst in you, are often trying to hide the worst in themselves!* Fearful people think you are too naive or blind to see your own way. Your wisdom is inferior to theirs. They know more than you or obviously you would have the same concerns as they do.

My pastor, Dr. Charles Stanley, has a term for these fearful people. He calls them, "back to Egypt people." When the Israelites first saw giants dwelling in the Promised Land, they wanted to go back to Egypt, where they had been slaves—because it was familiar. Wanting the known, while fearing the unknown, keeps you in bondage. Trust God to walk with you and conquer the giants that keep you from dwelling peacefully in your own "Promised Land." (You will learn in the S section that the Promise Land for the New Testament believer is rest—a condition not a location.)

The Drinkers

Many people, riddled with fear, cope by drinking alcohol. Their drinking is the infamous "white elephant in the room."

I'm sure you've been around people whose tongues gets looser and a little sharper, once they've consumed their second drink. That's when their inhibitions, along with their manners, go out the window. "Hello," Mr. and Mrs. Nasty have arrived.

These individuals never think their drinking is a problem. It's always you. You're the prude—the *kill-joy* or the *nervous Nellie*. They couldn't possibly have had too much to drink. They've been drinking for years, and they handle their liquor superbly—yeah, right! Well, forget sleep when these people are around. I hope you don't have one of these people in your intimate circle, but sadly millions do.

Concerning alcohol, the unfortunate truth is there is a line and once you cross it, you can never go back. Who knows where that ominous line is for each individual—in becoming an alcoholic?

The Dry Drunk

The more subtle and problematic person, however, is the dry drunk. These folks understand the term "white elephant in the room," but ironically, they inevitably project it onto you. The real granddaddy of all "white elephants" is the dry drunk's fear that feeds their controlling and judgmental behavior. These people—and maybe it's you—abstain from drinking, but they are not fully sober. Why? Because the fear that led them to drink in the first place is still their constant companion.

These individuals run around like the town crier, worrying about this and that—allowing their fear to turn them inside out—because in their subconscious mind, if they don't control everything (including you and your choices), they might drink again. As a form of cross-addiction—since they haven't dealt with what caused them to drink in the first place—many of these people are chain smokers. Letting go of fear is a crucial factor in overcoming addictions. Without a leg to stand on, surprisingly, these heavy ladened souls can be some of the most judgmental people you will ever encounter.

If you are a free person, living by faith—and have not bowed your knee to the "god of fear"—you'd be wise to realize fear-ridden people can never be your equal. You can love them, pray for them and even enjoy them to some degree, but if you are looking for advice concerning a relationship or some other matter, you can never go to them for wise counsel. They may be street-wise and can share some of their concerns, but usually they throw the baby out with the bath water. They are "all or nothing" types.

Unfortunately, they have self-medicated their pain for so long—failing to develop in certain areas—that they do not possess the maturity for giving wise, balanced counsel. *"Faithful are the wounds of a friend,"* the Bible tells us, but you need someone that understands how to tell you the truth in love—not in judgment, shrouded in condemnation—all of which are rooted in fear.

Judgmental people

Judgmental people rarely see the pain they cause others and the sleep robbers that they really are. *And*, they get it wrong more often than not. Here's the bottom line. We all struggle with this, but you and I as humans, are terrible at judging. Leave it to God. I am referring to the condemning aspects of judgement. These judging types need to be humble and look at their own stuff. Judgment is a relationship divider. It is a connection killer. Condemnation isolates and according to, Chris Williams, MA, LMFT, it creates a Petri dish for the very sin to grow that is under scrutiny by these holier than thou types.

Perhaps you can relate to the following scenario, as told by a well known pastor's wife:

Some of you are mothers, so you know what it is like to ask

your children to clean up their rooms. Imagine one day, after making such a request, you hear bantering between two children who share a room, until fighting inevitably breaks out and the younger child starts to cry. You go into the room to investigate what you already know to be true. The younger child is crying and full of drama, as he points to his older brother.

"He punched me!"

Your response is like a robot, as you turn to the older child. "What did you do?"

Full of justification, the oldest tells you, "He wouldn't clean up!"

But as you look around the room, you notice the older brother has not made his bed, nor has he gathered his clothes off the floor, to hang them in the closet. Immediately, you have to explain to this child, "You are not the parent. You take care of your assignment and I will handle your brother."

God doesn't need you or me to be the Holy Spirit. Talk to the Father about what concerns you in others. Ask Him to whisper to them what you are shouting. See if they don't respond to God's whispers rather than your shouting.

Nurses are often "rescuers" by nature, so I've met a few of these judgmental people along the way. Can you tell? They get a little carried away and are great at destructive criticism—but not constructive criticism. Instead of killing the fly on your forehead with a fly swatter, they whack you with a sledgehammer. The irony of it all, is that the very person you once helped—by extending to them grace rather than judgment—can in turn, become the one whacking you with the sledgehammer of judgment during your difficult season. Judgmental people will rob you blind in the sleep department, keeping you totally sleep deprived—but they need grace and forgiveness just like we all do.

Thankfully, these people can slowly, but surely change. It's rare but it does happen. They need a steady diet of God's Word, to help them mature, as well as grace and forgiveness, along with a change of friends that can confront their fear mongering and judgmental thinking in a loving consistent way. I have been privileged to see it work and know that when you are willing to change, you can.

Become a Person of Grace

Allow me to share with you, one of my all-time favorite stories as told by Steve Arterburn of New Life Ministries.

One day an unfortunate man falls into a hole and begins yelling for help. Eventually a physician comes by, writes a prescription, tosses it down to the man and tells him to call his office for an appointment. The physician begins to whistle a catchy tune and goes on his merry way. Next an attorney shows up, drops his business card down the hole and tells him to call his secretary to schedule some time on his calendar, as he scurries off to chase a passing ambulance with a deafening siren.

The man is dumb-founded. "How incredulous are these people?" he ponders to himself.

Then the unthinkable happens. His best friend, comes by and hears him yelling. So the friend immediately jumps down into the hole to help him. Now the man is totaling beside himself. "Why did you jump in this hole? I need help. You can't help me if you are stuck down here with me?"

The friend kindly says, "I fell in this hole last week and I know the way out."

When I heard this story, I told myself, "Never forget the moral of this story and it's powerful take away."

You'll never be a person of grace if you don't show humility to those that you are tempted to judge.

One thing I do that gives me grace for fearful people is to remember how I once lived as an insomniac, in fear. Have you ever asked yourself, "What's the worst thing that can happen? And then it happens, but somehow you're okay? I was so afraid I was going to lose my job. One day, that actually happened, but the Lord provided me with a job the very next week. I didn't even have time to worry because the competition called me the day I lost my job and asked me to come work for them. Sadly, since that particular job loss there have been several others due to market changes in my industry, but I have always been able to pay my bills. God has always provided for me.

I also lived with the fear my dad would die. He seemed to be so accident-prone and gave us so many scares—like sliding down the mountain on his tractor while bush hogging. In addition, he had allergies that required multiple surgeries for nasal polyps. When that dreaded moment finally came, my sister's rare phone call revealed that my dad would be leaving us soon.

She told me, "You need to come home. Dad's been diagnosed with a Glioblastoma." Two months later, he passed away. At the pronouncement of the most dreaded of all my anticipated moments—up to that point in my life—I experienced a peace that is not of this world. It was beyond my comprehension.

Perfect Provision

Corrie ten Boom, a Holocaust survivor and famous author, is known to have shared an experience with her father. She was scheduled to go on a train ride and was worried that her father had not yet given her the ticket for their trip. When she expressed her concern, her father lovingly told her, "When you need it, you will have it."

Your Heavenly Father is intimately acquainted with each and every need you have. Just like Corrie's train ticket—whatever you need—your Heavenly Father has already provided for that need. His provision may not be what you think it should be, or in the way you think it should be, but He who sees all and knows all, provides perfectly for you. This is why you can sleep in peace.

Worry slanders the character of God. You wouldn't want a child of yours telling their school teacher, "I'm afraid my parents aren't going to take care of me tonight. I hope they feed me. They have all of my life, but I don't know. What if they don't feed me tonight?"

As a child of God, Your Heavenly Father always provides above and beyond your needs, if you trust Him and allow Him to do so. All He asks is that you believe Him. The Bible tells us that faith comes by hearing the Word of God. If you struggle with fear, start reading the Book of Psalms. Every time you see the word "trust," circle it with a red pen. Then go back and re-read all the verses circled in red. See if your faith doesn't increase and your fear start to diminish. Feed your faith; starve your fear and enjoy lots of Zzz's.

Perfect love casts out all fear

Ultimately, I lost all fear in my life when I received the revelation of how much God loves me. Perfect love casts out all fear. Being so riddled with fear, at one point in my life, I developed Grave's disease. That was my wake up call. In order to reclaim my health, on a daily basis, I started reciting Joseph Prince's mantra: *"I live as a little child of God, carefree, stress free, worry free."* It got down in my soul, and I am free of fear. Knowing how much He loves me, allows me to sleep like a baby. I don't lose sleep because of fear, and I haven't in years.

1 John 4:18 tells us: *There is no fear in love; but perfect love casts out fear, because fear involves punishment, and the one who fears is not perfected in love.* Bill and Gloria Gaither know this truth and have captured it in a beautiful song called, I am Loved. See the chorus from their song below:

I am loved, I am loved
I can risk loving you
For the One who knows me best
Loves me most
I am loved you are loved
Won't you please take my hand
We are free to love each other
We are loved

Once you know how much God loves you, you become very comfortable in your own skin and you are able to focus on others not just yourself. You attract like-minded people. That is when life really gets good. That is truly the sweet spot and sleep comes easily.

Iron Sharpening Iron

There's a thin line between faith and foolishness. You may be someone or know someone who is living on the edge and calling it faith. A friend who is generally peaceful—but has a check in their spirit concerning some aspect of your life—may have a word of caution or a word of wisdom for you. This is someone you should give pause to and hear them out, because they are not driven by fear and condemnation but they are driven by love. These friends genuinely have your best interest at heart.

Keep these people in your life at all cost. They are rare and precious. God uses them to help you with your blind spots. I have a dear, forever friend like this. She is one of my most precious treasures. I tell her often that she is fine china.

The Scriptures speak of iron sharpening iron. If you are truly associating with healthy people, you will still have clashes and differences of opinion. But as long as there is mutual respect and a true interest in conflict resolution, then both parties can grow and become sharper individuals. When someone fails to see the other person's perspective, and always has to be right, that is not a person you need in your inner circle—unless he or she is willing to change, which would most likely require a Damascus Road experience.

Better to Love and Lose, Than Never Love

I have often wondered why some people come along who seem like they might be a life-partner, but in the end they don't make the cut. Many times, it's a result of ignoring your initial wisdom or the warning signs along the way—but not always. Not only can love be blind, but it can also be stubborn.

Perhaps you can relate to this. In some rare circumstances, God uses a relationship that ends in a break up to add iron to your character. It makes you more universal and helps you relate to all the broken-hearted people with whom you come in contact.

When it comes to love, if all you see is the gold fairy-dust, like Cinderella waiting for her prince to bring her the left-behind glass slipper, then . . . *real sorrow will be too unpoetic for you. The gold is but a vision, but the iron is an experience. The chain which unites you and me to humanity must be an iron chain. That touch of nature, which makes the world akin, is not joy, but sorrow; gold is partial but iron is universal*—George Mattheson.

"When God gives us a dream lined with gold, much like He gave Joseph in the Bible, by the time the dream enters our soul through experience, the gold becomes iron." (*Streams in the Desert*, Volume 1, September 8th, Mrs. Charles Cowman).

Relationships help us grow and yet, life gets messy. If you are self-protecting to a fault, you may not find love. Get out there and live, but set boundaries and apply wisdom. Perhaps you have heard it said, "It is better to have loved and lost, than to never have loved at all." If a relationship that you gave your heart and soul to does not work, you can still walk away a richer person—because God can use the experience to enlarge your soul through suffering. He can take the gold from all the hopes and dreams you had for that relationship and turn it into iron, which only happens when He enlarges your soul. Mrs. Cowman tells us, God doesn't do this by freeing you *from* suffering, but by freeing you *through* suffering.

Professional Help through Counseling

Be teachable and ask God to reveal your blind spots. The Bible tells us wisdom can be found in a multitude of counselors. Just make sure they haven't been poisoned by fear mongers before you jump on their bandwagon and take their advice.

Concerning ethical matters, it is wise to go to a professional counselor so that people don't betray or slander you in these situations. Talking to a qualified counselor avoids a land mine of problems, as friends may begin to feel overburdened or accuse you of taking advantage of them. In truth, some people mean well, they just don't have the maturity or faith to walk with you through your dilemma.

A word of caution: know your audience before you share with them. Again, these situations often call for a trained counselor to avoid unnecessary drama and more loss of sleep.

Perhaps the offense is from a spouse, a child or another family member. These dynamics are often complicated. Professional help, through the church or the community, may be necessary. Be gentle with yourself. Do whatever it takes to talk it out. Otherwise, you may be up at night for long periods of time, with disparaging thoughts and hurt emotions—robbing you of needed sleep. In addition to finding support, it is very important to journal during this season. You need the emotional catharsis. Do not take these emotions to bed with you.

Unforgiving People

Unforgiving, punitive people have no place in your life, especially concerning petty matters. When you make a mistake—whether innocent or intentional, or you experience a common misunderstanding but genuinely apologize—the other person needs to accept your apology, for your sake and theirs. Healthy people know this and act accordingly.

There will always be petty, unreasonable people. Sometimes, you just have to walk away. In situations where you can't cut ties, because they are family, a coworker or there is some other circumstance involved, take pity on their unforgiving souls. They have poured a poisonous drink, with the intent of serving it to you—all the while, they are the ones who end up drinking the cup of bitterness, as a result of their own unwillingness to forgive.

Always forgive. You only hurt yourself if you don't. Do whatever it takes to release the offense to God. Learn to forgive as quickly as possible. You only hurt yourself by holding a grudge. It physically affects you and causes disease.

If there is something bothering you—to the point that you can't sleep—entailing unresolved conflict with another person, write them a letter, whether they are dead or alive. Obviously, you can't mail a dead person a letter—and sometimes, you don't know where to send the letter if you have lost touch. It doesn't even matter if you send the letter. What does matter is that you finally get what's bothering you out of your system and out of your head—even if it's just on a piece of paper.

Now—maybe you can sleep! Once you are fresh, and you have given it some time, you can decide whether or not you want to mail the letter or send the email.

Misunderstandings

Nothing is more gut-wrenching than a good ole' fashioned misunderstanding. Talk about something that will keep you up all night—that will do it.

Misunderstandings are deeply painful, but they are going to happen. They are part of the human experience. These awful incidences can blindside you and change the trajectory of a friendship forever. But God is never caught off guard or surprised by these unfortunate scenarios. He sees them coming, long before you do. He is there to remind you that He is the most misunderstood Person of all. He feels your pain and loves to comfort you in trying times. Learn to hand Him your messes while you rest, knowing He will make them work for your good, if you love Him and are called according to His purpose.

Sometimes, you get caught between friends and are pulled in diametrically opposing directions. These situations call for a great deal of careful communication. Bring as much clarity to the matter as possible, by confessing your true motives. Behaviors are misleading, and people can draw all kinds of wrong conclusions. Have open, honest dialogue so that everyone is clear about what happened. This will prevent assumptions from running amuck.

I am reminded of the behavioral science teacher, who quizzed his students about a mouse's behavior that was free to roam around in a box. He wanted the students to observe the mouse's behavior and then tell him what motivated the mouse to demonstrate a particular behavior. The majority of the students decided the mouse was hungry, since he kept going to the edge of the box, in what looked like, an attempt to escape and get to the tray of food on the other side of the box. But the real reason this mouse kept walking into the walls was due to the simple fact, he was totally blind. The food in the tray was fake with no real aroma, so the mouse didn't even know there was anything remotely like food on the outside of the box. The blind mouse was actually orienting himself to his surroundings.

So often, things are not at all what they seem to be. When you observe someone's behavior without knowing the motive, you can really misread the entire situation and vice versa. When others judge your behavior without knowing your motive, they, too, can draw a wrong conclusion.

Again, letter writing is so important when it comes to resolving convoluted issues. When you are losing sleep over personality clashes and misunderstandings, letters can help you get closure, as well as some Zzz's.

Getting Clarity Helps You Get Your Zzz's

Dennis Prager, an author, speaker and radio talk host, is the king of clarity. He points out, it's not always that you want people to agree with you. Rather, it's that you want them to be clear about what the disagreement is. It takes good communication to tease this out because so many people project their own junk onto you, so that the whole issue gets muddled. In the end, whatever initially caused your disagreement may be miles away from the controversial issue at hand.

How many times have you thought a conflict was about X only to find out you were really arguing about Y? Sometimes, bringing clarity to a situation allows sleep to come more quickly, even if you still disagree with one another. All you really want in the end is for your perspective to be heard, understood, and validated—not necessarily embraced. Closure is often just the cure you need for insomnia. Learn to get closure as you go through life, so that you avoid imaginary conversations in your head—wishing you had clarified a matter.

Even when two people are deeply in love, they can view the same scenario and see it from diametrically opposing viewpoints. Two Christians serving the same Lord, both deeply committed to His kingdom principles, can look at the same situation and see it very differently. That's one of the reasons why we have denominations within Christianity.

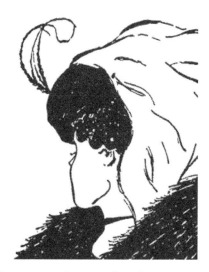

Look at the picture above. What do you see? An old woman or a young woman? The young woman has her jaw-line turned to the side with a choker around her neck. The old woman's nose is the young woman's jaw-line and chin, while the choker on the young woman is the old woman's mouth. Remember, there are at least two sides to every situation. There's not just one right viewpoint in most circumstances. It's not just how you see it; others have their perspective, too. Always be respectful of the other viewpoint. The exception to this, is man's viewpoint against God's viewpoint! His Word is final.

The Emery Boards

When you choose to invite healthy people into your inner circle, you have a head start on peaceful sleep. However, this fallen world is full of shady characters. There will always be plenty of opportunities to rub elbows with people who don't have your best interest in mind.

In her book, *The Best Is Yet to Come*, Ann Platz uses the term "sandpaper" people to describe the difficult types—the unbearable people in your life. These are the ones who walk out of a room, after they have thrown a hand grenade. When they return, they want to know who made the mess and what's wrong with everyone.

Whether these challenging people come in and out of your life for a season, or you are stuck with them for life—because they are perhaps family—seek God's wisdom before you confront them in love. Set firm boundaries around them. Take the emotion out of your voice, and be very matter of fact with them. When you respond in a way that demands their respect, you'll be able to hit the pillow with a fighting chance of falling asleep—and hopefully stay asleep throughout the night.

According to Ann Platz, "God, who is building His tabernacle in your heart, has a reason for every person He permits to touch your life. Even the 'sandpaper' people are designed for a purpose—to smooth the rough surfaces of your spirit and shape you for something the Lord has for you to do or to be. These people are extremely important: they can teach you valuable lessons—if you let them."

Think of your soul—character or personality—being shaped into Christ-likeness by these "sand paper people." Just as your nails are shaped by an emery board or finger nail file during a manicure, God is shaping you to be more like Christ in all you say, do and think.

The Netty Hearts

I recently heard the gifted Bible teacher, Beth Moore, deliver an extraordinary teaching on the matter of "netty hearts." You and I can have a netty heart and get trapped in difficult situations. The more we struggle, trying to get out of the net, the more tangled we become. We find ourselves in a real mess. You are already in a net, if you find yourself saying, "I never saw this coming. I have no idea how I got in this mess, and I can't imagine my life coming to this!"

With eyes wide open, you can find yourself in some very bad messes by willingly entering into questionable relationships. Conversely, you can also fall into terrible situations where you had no fore-warning. The enemy knows how to set traps for you that take you by complete surprise. Proverbs 1:17 (NIV) warns: *"How useless to spread a net where every bird can see it!"*

In addition to possibly possessing your own netty heart, you can also meet people with netty hearts that blind-side you. As you journey through life—like a net trap camouflaged in the jungle—out of nowhere, you can step into a trap set for you by the enemy. If you get caught in a relationship net, which turns out to be the challenge of a lifetime, you may need outside help to extricate yourself from the bondage. The Word tells us, in Psalms 25:15, *"My eyes are continually toward the Lord, for He will pluck my feet out of the net."*

Think of the word "pluck" and the concept of plucking your eyebrows. The Lord delivers you from netty relationships by plucking you out of the net—just like you tweeze stray hairs from the landscape of your perfectly manicured eyebrows.

Sometimes, it's impossible to know if you have the netty heart, or if the other person has the netty heart. Perhaps both of you do. When relationships are about *being held captive* to one another, this is a stronghold, and it is not of God. Cry out to Him to pluck you out of the net. Allow Him to re-establish you to a position of freedom. When you do this, He will un-tangle you, and He will do it in an unforeseen way. Once you are free, you will be able to sleep in peace.

The Princess and the Pea

A final word concerning overly sensitive people that rob you of sleep. Think of the childhood fairy-tale, the Princess and the Pea. The story unfolds with a young prince coming to his mother to announce he has found his true love. The Queen knows that she must determine if the girl is truly a princess, so she decides to test the young lady. The Queen invites her to stay for a night at the castle. After a royal dinner, held in her honor, the Queen escorts the princess to her room for the night.

The Queen has arranged for the princess to sleep on an outrageous stack of mattresses. But little does anyone know, the Queen has placed a tiny pea under the mattress at the bottom of the pile. She knows that if this girl is a real princess, she'll be so sensitive that she will awaken and present herself the next day, black and blue from the pea placed beneath the mattresses.

The following morning, the princess, exhausted from tossing and turning throughout the night, is black and blue, and the Queen instantly knows that her son has found a true princess—a young lady possessing true sensitivity.

If you have a princess in your world, get ready for some fun. Life is just too hard and unbearable for them. Dealing with them is real work, and there are not enough words to tell you how much sleep you will lose. Their goal is to train you to behave in such a way that you don't upset them. If one of these sensitive types happens to be a part of your life, making you constantly tippy toe around them, you have my deepest sympathy. Get ready to spend your days walking on egg shells. These control freaks get away with murder—because no one wants to upset them.

You may know these sensitive types by the common millennial term, "snowflakes." They are taking over the world. Be gracious and compassionate with them but firm. Set boundaries. Don't be manipulated by these sensitive ones or you will be in the hospital from sleep deprivation. This bears repeating from the U section: We need to love them while we toughen them up—for their own good and the overall good of society!

Forever Friends

People come and go—in and out of our lives—like revolving doors. When a season closes, and someone fulfills their purpose in your life, or vice versa, let them go, but always with a blessing. If you are blessed enough to have a great friend, be a good friend, and enjoy each other immensely. At night when you count, not sheep, but your Zzz's and your blessings, count these friends twice because they are a double blessing. Ask God to give you good friends, when you are in need, and He will amaze you. He will give you forever friends.

I'm reminded of a song, released during my college years, when I was working as a summer camp counselor for young girls. So many treasured friends materialized during those three years at summer camp. The song was written by Michael W. Smith, and the words are simply beautiful:

"Friends"

Packing up the dreams God planted
In the fertile soil of you
I can't believe the hopes He's granted
Means a chapter of your life is through

But we'll keep you close as always
It won't even seem you've gone
'Cause our hearts in big and small ways
Will keep the love that keeps us strong

And friends are friends forever
If the Lord's the Lord of them
And a friend will not say never
'Cause the welcome will not end

Though it's hard to let you go
in the Father's hands we know
That a lifetime's not too long
To live as friends

With the faith and love God's given
Springing from the hope we know
We will pray the joy you live in
Is the strength that now you show

We'll keep you close as always
It won't even seem you've gone
'Cause our hearts in big and small ways
Will keep the love that keeps us strong

And friends are friends forever
If the Lord's the Lord of them
And a friend will not say never
'Cause the welcome will not end

Though it's hard to let you go
In the Father's hands we know
That a lifetime's not too long
To live as friends

There is only one relationship I can recommend to you that will ultimately satisfy you in every way—including sleep. A relationship with the One who created you and gave His life for you; He offers you the *exchanged life*—the most extravagant gift ever lavished on anyone. I want to offer you a relationship and fellowship with this awesome God. Note: This is a relationship not religion.

The Exchanged Life

Remember when our fun, fictitious, *Holiday* friend, Amanda, learned that Iris wanted to do a house swap? The idea of a two-week getaway fascinated Amanda and, in no time, the girls switched houses with each other. The results were course-correcting and life changing. As you watch the movie, you see each character move away from toxic people to happy, wholesome ones. Think of it! You and I have the opportunity for an even greater exchange with our Creator.

Jesus Christ offered Himself as the sacrificial Lamb to bear all that is wrong, disappointing or flawed in you. Your fallen nature and selfishness were taken and projected onto Him. In exchange, He credited to you, His perfect love and His right standing with the Father—God's righteousness, along with all His glorious riches.

There is nothing you can imagine or believe you have need of that Jesus has not provided. It's an unbelievable package of benefits that He so willingly longs to bestow on you. His sacrifice was—and is—complete and whole.

Once you really understand and embrace the *exchanged life,* sleep is sure to ensue. He, who never slumbers, works the nightshift so you don't have to do anything but sleep. Give Him your insomnia, and He will give you sweet sleep—a minuscule fraction of the overall exchange.

Perhaps you also need to give Him your messy, tangled life. How about relinquishing your fear of losing control, which can manifest itself in an overbearing, controlling and judgmental disposition? Give your loving Heavenly Father your fallen sin nature—your regret, guilt, disease, poverty, shame, and bondage. In exchange, He will give you righteousness, forgiveness, pardon, health, abundant life, freedom, supply, restorative sleep . . . and His "gift list" goes on and on.

When you understand what Christ did for you, you will no longer remain in bondage in any area of your life. You will demand your freedom. Even though Christ won the victory—at a tremendous cost that you can't begin to fathom—you could still be living in bondage, even as a believer. Why is this so? Despite the fact that Jesus purchased you with an outlandish blood-bought price, Satan is still squatting on the property of freedom that God has given you.

Satan hates you, and he wants you in bondage. He will stop

at nothing to rob you of what Jesus has provided. But once you learn what happened on the cross, you can be free. You have to serve Satan his eviction papers. Only you, however, can make him leave. You must command him to go in Jesus' name. You must command the chains of bondage to fall off. Satan and his lies, bondage, darkness, vices, addictions, all have to leave. Jesus has done all that is needed to free you and me. Whenever Satan shows up, we have to put on our armor (Ephesians 6:13-18) and take authority over him, in Jesus name— and make him go!

Amanda got the short end of the stick, when it came to her house swap. Iris' cottage didn't quite compare to Amanda's beautiful home in sunny LA. The exchange that I'm introducing to you is in no way fair either. You receive unbelievable blessings in exchange for all of your curses.

The *great exchange* that took place on the Cross is available to you today by simply praying this heartfelt prayer:

The Exchanged Life Prayer

Lord Jesus,
I know I am a sinner.
No matter how good of a person I think I am,
It does not meet Your standard of perfection and holiness.
Please forgive me of my sins.
I believe You shed Your blood for me,
Because You love me more than I can possibly comprehend.
You lavishly paid for my sins and rescued
me from poverty, fear, disease, and insomnia.
You have given me eternal life and a future and a hope.
Please take over my life and allow
Your Spirit to dwell within me.
I trust and follow You as my Lord and Savior.
Guide my life and help me do Your will.
Impart to me Your abundant life.

Please send me friends that know You and will help me grow
In my walk with You, so I can enjoy sweet sleep
and fulfill my destiny.
Help me take care of myself,
so I can be available to help others along the way.
In Your name, the name above all names, I ask this,
Amen.

RELIGION

Religion is a two-edged sword. For all the good it provides, it also offers an equal and opposing downside. I've just explained what it means to have a personal relationship with God through faith in Jesus Christ. But it's important to note that "religion" is different than a personal relationship with Jesus. Keep reading!

Religion on a Global Scale Can Keep You Up at Night

If life wasn't already difficult enough, you now face the added burden of possible terror attacks—with wars about to break out all over the globe. The Bible is quite clear that, in this fallen world, there will always be wars and rumors of war. Matthew 24:6 says, *"And you shall hear of wars and rumors of war: see that you be not troubled: for all these things must come to pass, but the end is not yet."*

As beneficial as religion can be in helping society find purpose and meaning to life, many of the wars around the world are due to extremist points of view about religion.

Most religious matters are not extreme. However, you've probably never heard of a terrorist who wasn't religious—whether it is a right-winged loon, bombing an abortion clinic or a Radical Islamic Jihadist beheading his victim. There is no way to imagine the suffering of the persecuted Church across the ocean, unless you have lived near it or been a part of it.

Examine religion, or the lack of religion, in your life to see if your worldview is keeping you up at night. Religion offers the hope that you will be reconciled to God, so that you can be in right standing with Him. However, religion itself will never ultimately do what it promises. It is a set of rules that must be followed to the letter of the law. It requires that you live under the law—knowing the law is completely unforgiving. Religion requires that in order to be in right standing with God, you must keep His law perfectly. Therefore, religion is man's feeble attempt at appeasing God. It is Mankind, in its fallen state, reaching up to a holy perfect God, attempting to reconcile the sinful nature of humanity.

I'm reminded of the dog that was locked up in a garage all day. Out of boredom, he chewed some wires on the boat parked in the garage. He had no idea what he had done, but when the owner came home, he took the dog straight to the vet and had him put to sleep. This is a picture of how unforgiving the law is.

But picture a similar scene differently, when grace is added. In the next scenario, while the dog is in the house—waiting for his master to return—his canine nose catches a whiff of something interesting in the trash. Once the master returns, he discovers trash all over the kitchen floor. Tapping the dog on the backside with a newspaper to teach him not to do this, the master then cleans up the mess, because he understands the limits of his dog. The master knows that dogs can never clean up their messes.

The Ten Commandments were written to show that you and I will never be able to keep these laws—not 100% of the time. We have all sinned and fallen short, missing the mark in one way or another—no matter how hard you and I try. Therefore, you and I need a Savior.

Just as you have already read in the relationship section, Jesus desires a relationship with you. Forget about performing for Him and keeping the law. He wants you to get out of the kitchen. Stop preparing the meal and just come, sit, and dine at the table He has prepared for you. Relax and rest in His grace. Ask Him to be your Lord and Savior. Exchange your sin—your mess—for His forgiveness. Do this and start enjoying your life.

Get off the religious treadmill—and just breathe! Allow Jesus to love you. As you begin to rest in His love, you'll be empowered to live the Christian life effortlessly. You'll be fruitful—not just busy. Otherwise, you will be back on the religious treadmill of working and performing—becoming exhausted by the effort.

How do you do this? Pray the Exchanged Life Prayer, provided for you at the end of the relationship portion of this section or see Appendix A. Get a Bible and read a passage from it every day. It is the Word of God that will help you stay in perfect peace, as you build a relationship with Him. Find a Bible-believing church that welcomes you and teaches you the Christian faith. Ask God to lead you to the right house of worship.

When people get this wrong—thinking they have to be perfect for God—they unknowingly reject Him. This creates all kinds of faulty conclusions. Some of the most severely fragile, and tragically insecure people are attracted to fringe ideologies that promote over the top acts "for God." Extremist groups know this and prey on weak individuals to accomplish their evil deeds, doing it in the name of their "god"—not the one true God. This is how recruiting and radicalization works for Radical Islam.

Perhaps you can't sleep because you're worried about these destructive ideologies. If you've lived long enough, you can probably recall where you were, and what you were doing, when the 9/11 terror attacks occurred.

More recently, people remember watching round-the-clock coverage of the events in both Paris and Nice, France, as well as in Brussels. The attack on our own soil, in Orlando, Florida, was also devastating. Terrorism is escalating throughout Europe—not to mention the ongoing nightmares happening in Israel. With no real end in sight, we all have to make peace with the temptation to be crippled by fear. This is the purpose of terrorism. They want you to live in fear, adversely affecting your sleep in a major way.

Psalm 91, a classic Scripture, is often the chosen text to assail brewing fears related to terror attacks. The entire chapter is very comforting, but quoting Psalm 91:1, as you are calling upon God for help in time of trouble, is God's 9-1-1 for distressed callers.

Whenever you need to calm your fears—concerning terrorism, soaring crime rates, dangerous newly discovered viruses, increasing numbers of earthquakes, or any other worry—meditate on this beautiful Scripture. It will calm your soul and help you sleep. Be especially mindful of verse *five, regarding matters of sleep.

Psalm 91
New American Standard Bible (NASB)

*He who dwells in the shelter of the Most High
Will abide in the shadow of the Almighty.
I will say to the Lord, "My refuge and my fortress,
My God, in whom, I trust!"
For it is He who delivers you from the snare of the trapper
And from the deadly pestilence.
He will cover you with His pinions,
And under His wings you may seek refuge;
His faithfulness is a shield and a bulwark.*
***You will not be afraid of the terror by night,
Or the arrow that flies by day;***
*Of the pestilence that stalks in darkness,
Or of the destruction that lays waste at noon.*

A thousand may fall at your side
And ten thousand at your right hand,
But it shall not approach you.
You will only look on with your eyes
And see the recompense of the wicked.
For you have made the Lord, my refuge,
Even the Most High, your dwelling-place.
No evil will befall you,
Nor will any plague come near your tent.
For He will give His angels charge concerning you,
To guard you in all of your ways.
They will bear you up in their hands,
That you do not strike your foot against a stone.
You will tread upon the lion and the cobra,
The young lion and the serpent you will trample down.
"Because he has loved Me, therefore I will deliver him;
I will set him securely on high
because he has known My name."
"He will call upon Me and I will answer him;
I will be with him in trouble;
I will rescue him and honor him."
"With long life I will satisfy him
And let him see My salvation."

John 16:33 conveys that you will have trouble in this world, because it is fallen, but He tells you—you can overcome. Without becoming exhaustive, I believe when you are in Christ, you are encapsulated and divinely shielded, even in the midst of calamity and death.

I think of being in my car while going through the automated car wash. Because the car has to be in neutral, all I can do is sit in the car while the machines and the tracking for the wheels escort me through all the commotion. The swirling mops, and vicious soapy water would physically harm me and bring havoc to my safety, if I were not safe inside the car. But when all is said and done, my outlook and my mode of transportation, as I journey through life are brighter and cleaner having gone through the car wash countless times. I am better for the experience but only because I was protected inside the car.

Just like being safely inside your vehicle throughout the entire car wash at the car spa, when trouble assails and you are flooded with the cares of this world, rest knowing you are hidden in Christ. Even in death, He is with you, so you have nothing to fear. His angels encamp around you. Because death is inevitable for all of us, you can say in total confidence, when your final moment comes, *"I walk through the valley of the shadow of death, and I will fear no evil,"* because you know He covers you—when you are in Christ.

Religious Scenarios Closer to Home Can Keep you up at Night

On a less global scale, there are plenty of scenarios—within the religious world—that are quite unsettling. Although some of the most loving people can be found in Christian circles, as it should be—some of the meanest men and women you'll ever meet are at church. Mean girls aren't just in high school! The church is a healing place for the sick, but don't be surprised if you get hurt there. Perhaps you have heard this adage, "Hurt people, hurt people." I hope you are not someone who is inflicting some of the pain.

Think of the Christian congregation as being comprised of caterpillars and butterflies. Everyone is at a different stage in their faith journey. Some believers are more mature than others. Some are new caterpillars, some are cocooning, and others have gone through metamorphosis, so they've become butterflies. This metamorphosis for a believer is known as the process of sanctification. You are being changed from glory to glory. The Bible tells us, if you are in relationship with Christ, you will change for the better. People change differently— some slowly, while others do it more quickly. So, cut people some slack. You never know what stage of growth they are in.

Ask God to lead you to butterflies in the body of Christ— mature Christians that understand the message of grace. They can help you, mentor you and teach you how to grow in your walk with God. If you are a butterfly, look for ways to help caterpillars along the way.

There is no legitimate place for a clique at church. Make sure you create an atmosphere of inclusiveness. Be sensitive to others. Keep your radar up for situations where you can extend yourself, going the extra mile. Boundaries are needed at church, however, but always communicate the truth, in love.

The Word Changes You so You Can Keep the Peace

Nothing helps me sleep more than listening to Scripture lullabies www.scripture-lullabies.com or Scripture readings. Reading the Word changes your thoughts, but listening to the Word changes your emotions. At night, when you are worried, listen to audio Scripture on www.biblegateway.com. Close your eyes and let God's words calm you and diminish your worries. Do a trade with Him. Give Almighty God your cares and concerns and let Him bless you with sweet sleep.

"Casting all your anxiety on Him, because He cares for you"
(1 Peter 5:7).

"Be anxious for nothing,
but in everything by prayer and supplication
with thanksgiving let your requests be made known to God.
And the peace of God, which surpasses all comprehension,
will guard your hearts and your minds in Christ Jesus"
(Philippians 4:6-7).

What is keeping Amanda up at night?

On a day-to-day basis, Amanda is not concerned about terrorism, but there is a line in the movie where she refers to a terrorist—in the global sense of the word. During one of her rambling rants, she says, "Single women over the age of 35 are more likely to be killed by a terrorist than get married." Overall, she was completely free to worry about all sorts of things without ever being deterred by any real terrorist threats. Unfortunately, when you consider living with daily terror— like our Israeli friends do—this sure does provide perspective. It is amazing how quickly petty issues no longer matter, if you are running into a bomb shelter multiple times a day.

For Amanda, finding the answer to what was keeping her up at night boiled down to simply getting away from the rat race. Once she abandoned her work and everything familiar, she was able to quieten her mind. At that moment, she found someone she could love. Suddenly, sleep was no longer an issue, because her relationships and roles were no longer toxic. Making a concerted effort to remodel her life—in order to live her dream—required taking a big risk and a great deal of determination, as well as courage. If you remodel your life, so that you can finally get needed sleep, this will be required of you, as well.

In many cases, true insomnia is a spiritual problem. Although Amanda's insomnia was cured through the typical *reel* Hollywood cure—a dream relationship—in *real* life, when you have a relationship with the One who created you, you definitely sleep much better.

Just as Amanda doesn't demonstrate being religious, I'm not a religious person either. She is relational, and so I am. True Christianity is relational. It is not a religion.

The exchanged life is a personal faith walk with the One who created you and purchased you. If you give Him your worries and concerns, He will give you sweet sleep in return. Joseph Prince tells all of us to remain at rest. This is the secret to receiving God's best. If all I had was religion but no relationship, I would never sleep in peace.

The One who created you, also created sleep, and He's got the answers to your question, "What's keeping me up at night?"

You are now ready to move on to the spiritual side of sleep. You will discover some of God's truths to help you enjoy sanctified sleep—sleep that is set apart for His purposes. It's not just to rejuvenate your body and your soul, but also your spirit. As a triune being, you are a spirit with a soul in a body, designed to welcome sleep—a holy vesper to the close of your day—where dreams are meant to abound.

SLEEP Q-TIPS:

- Never carry anger to bed with you. If someone makes you angry, give it to God. Vengeance is His. He has your back. Trust Him. He will work it out for your good.

- Ask God to bring you genuine friends that don't rob you of precious sleep.

- Be a good friend and you will attract good friends. Look for like-minded people. People that don't keep you up at night.

- Forgive others quickly so you can sleep in peace.

- Live within your means. Less is more. Otherwise, you may toss and turn all night worrying.

- When it comes to sleep, use third stage thinking. Think long-term as you consider the consequences to yourself of not sleeping enough.

- Consider the cost to others when you don't sleep.

- If you are a caregiver to your loved one, suffering from sundowners due to dementia and they fall asleep in a chair, don't arouse them or try to get them to bed. Let them stay there and sleep as long as they will. You should take advantage of the situation and sleep while they sleep.

- Do something you love with your life. There are no "do overs" and you only get one go around. Hit the pillow knowing that you are living the life you wanted.

- Love your family and show them your love by spending quality time with them. Be a well rested family so that you can all be your best for each other.

- Friendships that are healthy, possess two great ingredients for sleep—peace and relaxation. People that put you at ease and breed peaceful, relaxing atmospheres, deserve front row seats in your life. These are the people that set you up to win so you drift off to dreamland in peace every night.

- Unhealthy friendships, riddled with fear, are manipulative, controlling and condemning. These relationships are toxic and will keep you up at night. At best, allow them to be balcony people in your life or perhaps you just need to boot them to the lobby so you have a fighting chance at sleep.

- To learn more about setting boundaries for all people but especially for the types that keep you up at night, read Henry Cloud's books, *Necessary Endings and Boundaries: When to Say Yes, How to Say No to Take Control of Your Life,* coauthored with John Townsend.

- To learn more about the harm and consequences of judging and condemning, as well as, how to stop the downward cycle that it breeds, read the book, *Without Rival,* authored by Lisa Bevere. You don't want to be a sleep-robber to anyone and no one needs to be robbing you of your Zzz's.

- Walk the line of love always as you set boundaries, remain firm but compassionate. This works on your sleep-life like a good mattress that is firm but soft.

- If you struggle with whether or not you believe in God, or if you have abandoned your faith, check out Andy Stanley's three part online series: *Who Needs God?* northpoint.org/messages/who-needs-god/. I can honestly tell you, if I had no relationship with our Lord or if all I had was religion but no relationship, I'd be an insomniac.

S: THE N.U.R.S.E. APPROACH TO RESTORATIVE SLEEP:

The Spiritual Side of Sleep—
Sanctified Sleep Set Apart for Dreams

Sleep-The Magic Carpet of Dreams

Sleep Soliloquy and Journaling—
Sleep Affirmations

Scripture Reading Played Audibly Induces Sleep

New Associations with Sleep and Sheep

The Shepherd Who Never
Sleeps So His lambs Can

True Shalom

Scriptures for Sleep and a Song for Sleep

THE SPIRITUAL SIDE OF SLEEP—SANCTIED SLEEP SET APART FOR DREAMS

Sleep has many benefits, most of which have already been addressed. There is one very special spiritual benefit to sleep, however, not yet mentioned. It's dreaming. Dreams can be profound and powerful, revealing important information from the subconscious to the conscious mind.

When sleeping soundly and restfully, it is quite natural to have your dreams direct you in ways your conscious mind would never entertain. Knotted, twisted thoughts untangle in dreams and communicate to you, at your subconscious level. A dream can help your mind get to the root of bewildering matters, such as, scrambled childhood memories or events that are blurred.

I believe, as you sleep, God finally gets you to rest so that He can do a deep work on your behalf—in your situations and circumstances. Sometimes, He gives you clues through your dreams, concerning certain matters that may need your immediate attention. Perhaps you need to make a course correction. Other times, He will give you encouragement through your dreams. This can help you settle the matter in your mind and help you determine that you are on the right track.

There are countless examples in the Scriptures where God uses dreams with His children to help them solve major problems. Daniel and Joseph are prime examples of men in the Bible who had prophetic and instructional dreams. They were also gifted at knowing and understanding the meaning of other people's dreams, as dream interpreters.

The late John Paul Jackson, author of *Understanding Dreams and Visions*, is the founder of Streams Ministries. He was an amazingly gifted, as well as an anointed dream interpreter. Therefore, he was my go-to-guy for my own dream interpretations. Thankfully, his television show, *Dreams and Mysteries*, still airs on Daystar and can also be seen on the Internet. Because of this, you and I are blessed with continuous access to an exhaustive wealth of his timeless wisdom and knowledge—concerning any and every possible aspect of dreams.

John Paul Jackson lists these 20 categories of dreams, divided into seven groupings:

Dreams to Reach Your Destiny
Prophetic and Revelatory Dreams, Calling Dreams, Courage Dreams, Direction Dreams, Invention Dreams, Word of Knowledge Dreams

Dreams to Change Your Path
Correction Dreams, Warning Dreams, Self-Condition Dreams

Dreams for Healing and Transformation
Healing Dreams, Deliverance Dreams, Flushing Dreams

Dreams from the Enemy
Dark Dreams, False Dreams, Fear Dreams

Dreams We Cause to Be Dreamed
Soul Dreams

Dreams to Train You in Spiritual Obedience
Spiritual Warfare, Intercession Dreams

Dreams Caused by Changes in Your Body
Chemical Dreams, Body Dreams

The dream categories overlap, so your dreams may fall into one or more of these groupings. Let's explore, at least, two of the categories.

First, **Dreams to Reach Your Destiny** are unique dreams that help you fulfill your calling in life. These dreams reveal information you could not have known naturally. Sometimes, they inform you of future events. These vivid dreams often consist of vibrant, bright colors and leave a spiritual residue that haunts you long after you awaken. This type of dream sticks in your mind, because the message is very important in helping you live out your divine purpose. All dreams in the 20 categories of Jackson's list, however, are classified as God dreams, but this category stands out over and above the other dream categories.

Second, **Dreams to Change Your Path**: This category of dreams tells you that something has to go—these dreams change the trajectory of your life's direction. There is something that is blocking your destiny from being fulfilled. The self-condition dream in this category, deals with your blind spots. Of all the dreams, this is the one classification that John Paul Jackson said people most frequently request for interpretation. It's as high as 80%, for obvious reasons. This dream equates to receiving a status report from your Heavenly Father about the difference between—where He wants you to be—and where you actually are.

Think of Amanda—our fictitious character from the movie, *Holiday*. She winds up thousands of miles from her home and totally remodels her life, when she makes just one simple, but profound, decision. She decides to deal with the pain of her insomnia caused by other extraneous issues. Once she chooses to jump off the treadmill of her out-of-balance life, she ends up changing her inner circle of friends and re-thinking her career. The results are stunningly satisfying.

A dream has the power to cause you to make one change, by which you find yourself fully awake to a whole new direction in life—but you have to be in tune with what you're dreaming. More importantly, for this to happen, you have to be asleep.

Allow me to illustrate this point.

A very important man in my life had a dream once. He dreamed he was in Israel running through an open field with land mines. His guide had to stop and tell him to leave his luggage. It was slowing him down and putting him in danger.

I met him at Starbucks the morning after his dream. As he

began to share the content of the dream, I knew his dream meant he was moving and he couldn't have anything in his life slowing him down. He had some things he needed to do for his family. I believe it was God's way of allowing me to be at peace with the decision. So dreams can speak to you, even if someone else dreams them. He was not sure about what to do, but I was able to encourage him to go, since I understood the dream's message.

If you are blessed with the ability to sleep uninterrupted, for about eight hours each night, you are supplying the basic favorable condition, necessary for dreaming to occur. There will probably be three phases of non-REM sleep throughout this time period. In the first stage of non-REM sleep, the eyes are closed, and there is no REM (Rapid Eye Movement). You'll barely be asleep, so you will still be easy to arouse. This stage lasts for 5–10 minutes.

The second phase of non-REM sleep continues to be a light state of sleep, but your body temperature drops, and your heart rate begins to slow down to around 60 beats a minute—all in preparation for deep sleep. This is why certain instrumental music with 60 beats a minute, helps to induce sleep. Essentially, the music and the pulse beat are in sync.

Third, the deep sleep phase of non-REM sleep is where restorative sleep occurs. To keep from prematurely aging, on average, you probably need much more sleep than you're getting. You actually need as much sleep as when you were younger. Sleep helps you experience rejuvenation and restoration. It also helps repair and regrow bone and muscle tissue, as well as, boost the immune system. If you are aroused during this phase, you'll feel disoriented, because this is a deep phase of sleep.

Once REM or dream sleep occurs, the first phase is about ten minutes and usually does not occur until 90 minutes into your sleep. As REM sleep comes and goes throughout the night, the duration of REM sleep lengthens to about four hours. The mind is very active during REM sleep. Therefore, at this juncture of sleep, your dreams can really be intense. This information was gathered from the National Institutes of Health and the National Sleep Foundation, as well as, the following article: http://www.webmd.com/sleep-disorders/guide/sleep-101.

Sadly, insomnia robs you of this heavenly aspect of sleep. So, you need to do everything in your power to set the stage for restorative sleep to return to you, so you can dream again.

The Magic Carpet of Dreams

In *Seeing the Voice of God*, Laura Harris Smith refers to sleep as the mattress of dreams, but I'm going to call sleep "the magic carpet" of dreams. Dreaming is a wonderful state of being, where gravity no longer matters. You can fly and do a host of things that the physical world limits. On "the magic carpet"—which is sleep—you can go anywhere in your dreams. You can even see loved ones or pets that have gone before you.

One of my all-time favorite dreams involves a visit from my little dog, Mickie. He died of cancer the week after Thanksgiving, in 2009. I was devastated because I had no warning. The following week I lost my job—another huge surprise. Immediately afterward, I was hired by the competition, but I was not supposed to start until the New Year, in January.

The new job proved to be unbearable—management was nothing less than a pit of hissing demons. You could not win with these people. They were foolish, insecure "wanna be's," with a Liberace management style. I was so stressed I could not sleep. One night, when it was 5:30 a. m., and I had not slept a wink, I prayed, "Lord, can You just let me sleep one hour?" I needed one hour of sweet sleep, at least, before my 8:00 a.m. daily call from Hell—with the hissing demons.

Somehow, I was able to drift off into a deep sleep. It was as though the minute sleep came, I was transported to Heaven. As I stood on a charming, neighborhood street aligned with rows of enchanted bungalows, showcasing the most pristine yards imaginable, I was awestruck. Low to the ground morning fog, mixed with a soft glow—from the promise of the rising sun—permeated the landscape. The brilliant, but muted, colors infusing the scenery was nothing I could describe. However, the peace and calm was as palpable and as evident as the fog I could see. In this dream, my neighbor who is still alive on planet earth came walking up to me, while holding my little dog in her arms. Mickie was perfect and completely adorable—just like the little eight-pound Pomeranian that left me.

I wanted to reach out and take him into my arms, but somehow I knew I couldn't have him. My neighbor was pleasant but never said a word. She communicated subtly—through my subconscious—that I couldn't have him. It was an inner knowing in my spirit.

With joy bubbling up inside of me, like a fountain, I exclaimed, "Mickie!"

My little fur baby replied in the sweetest voice, "Hi, Joni." As if to say, "Hi, Mama." Then he smiled.

One thing about Mickie, he had lost all but two of his canine teeth, while he was with me on earth. I had to allow the veterinarian to pull them because he was a rescue and his previous owner neglected his teeth. All of a sudden, when he smiled in the dream, he flashed a new set of gorgeous teeth— but they were beautiful veneer, human-like teeth. Then, he started talking to me in Hebrew, which I personally believe is the language of Heaven. I do not speak or understand it now—but I believe I will in Heaven.

All at once I awoke, feeling as though I had slept for days. I was invigorated by the dream—deep within my soul—because it was so affirming and healing. I knew my little Mickie was fine, and I would see him again. That dream put me in the best mood, but without that dream—I would have had a miserable day, due to sleep deprivation. It was one of the most precious experiences of my life.

Recently, I had some uncomfortable feelings towards a person due to some statements that bothered me. In other words, it was some *"I heard it through the grapevine"* stuff. I was hurt by it, until one night I had a dream. In the dream, our whole gang was in a little fifties diner, resembling one from a movie I recently watched. But the movie had a twist. It featured a modern day Jesus as part of the storyline.

There was no obvious person in my dream that would have been Jesus, but there was supernatural joy, pervading the atmosphere due to His presence. Throughout the dream, I kept my distance from the person that hurt me, until I was loading my plate—buffet style—when she reached past me and lovingly patted me on the back. Instantly, all the hurt left, and it has never returned. This was another dream that turned out to be a gift. I still have not seen her since the offense, but I believe it will be fine when I do. I am completely at peace with her because of my dream.

In dreams, you experience what you know instinctively, but are forced to suppress because of your demanding schedule. Sadly, even though you perceive something beneficial in your dream, often you don't pause and listen, because you're far too busy to hear. Sleep works to keep you alert during the day so you can be sharp, recognizing and resolving issues on the spot. But if you are sleep-deprived, this ability will be missing from your life.

Dreams allow you to revisit unresolved issues that go unnoticed throughout the day, thereby helping you avoid a host of problems. For example, if your mind tells you to pay the rent, but you forget in your busy-ness, that night while you sleep, your mind may alert you through a dream. Perhaps you dream that you are suddenly homeless. If you are tuned in to your dreams, you can heed the warning and avoid a late fee, by taking care of your rent in a timely manner. It's a minor issue compared to ending up homeless, as you were in the dream. Dreams often go over the top to get your attention.

John Paul Jackson, through the authorship of Michael Wise, helps you see the heart of God. Your Heavenly Father longs to lull you to sleep so you can commune, undistracted. The daily grind often crowds out His precious voice. Through dreams, He can warn you of dangers and concerns, much like a parent telling their child to hold hands on a busy side street or in a crowded parking lot. Your Heavenly Father often longs to encourage you through a dream—much like an earthly father who encourages his child when they learn to read a new word.

You have an omniscient Father who knows the future, and He is able to alert you, through your dreams, to future events that are going to happen—not just in your life but also in other people's lives. He wants to give you specific instructions. Perhaps He has creative solutions or a course correction in mind.

That is why journaling becomes so valuable—you don't want to miss His messages to you, through your dreams. Journaling causes you to reflect on all aspects of the dream, so you can respond to the dream accordingly.

SLEEP SOLILOQUY AND JOURNALING YOUR DREAMS

Laura Harris Smith says that you should write your dreams down upon awakening. If you can't take the time to journal them; at the very least, verbalize your dream out loud. Try to tell the content of the dream to someone, while it is still fresh on your mind.

Colors and symbols, as well as themes, are very important, so the longer you wait to record the dream or recite it, the chances of fabricating parts of it greatly increase, thereby compromising the real message of the dream and the integrity of the interpretation. In the past, I have actually told myself the dream in front of the mirror, but probably the best way is to record or video it on your cell phone or some other handheld device. You can transcribe the dream in your journal at a later date.

When journaling, if at all possible, document your dream immediately, when you first wake up. It is helpful to record:

- Recurring themes, colors, images and symbols
- Your feelings while you were dreaming
- How you felt upon awakening

According to Gayle Green, 60 million Americans can't sleep well. This is why sleep is such a hot topic in all aspects of today's society. I have even heard it touted that sleep is the new sex—meaning everyone's talking about sleep but no one is getting any sleep. It was intended from the beginning of time that you get plenty of Zzz's. However, if you are not sleeping, you are not alone. You need to do whatever you can to get restorative sleep. Be committed to getting enough sleep and enjoy the following enlightening facts, according to Laura Harris Smith:

- You spend one third of your life in bed.
- At age 75, you will have slept 25 years.
- It's scientifically proven that you have 16–36 dreams each night.
- In a lifetime you dream almost 1,000,000 dreams.

SPEAKING AFRMATIONS OF SLEEP EACH DAY

Hopefully, I've caused you to become excited about dreaming, and you'll be more interested in—not just sleeping—but sleeping soundly throughout the night, allowing "the magic carpet" of sleep to escort you to dreamland. One of the most important but frequently overlooked components in conquering insomnia is guarding the words you speak about your "sleep life."

If you go around saying:

"I can't sleep."
"I never sleep."
"I've never been able to sleep."
"I'm an insomniac!"

Change your words immediately!

Say only these words:

"Sleep loves me."
"I sleep like a baby."
"I am going to get a great night's sleep."
"My Heavenly Father protects my sleep."
"He gives me sweet sleep."

Words contain creative power. Words are life producing. The words you say really do matter. Guard your words. Speak sleep into your daily routine. All through the day, from this day forward, whether you have trouble with insomnia or not, let your words be filled with affirmations of sleep.

SCRIPTURE READING PLAYED AUDIBLY INDUCES SLEEP

You are a triune being made in the image of God. Your words are vitally important, but even more important are His Words.

Allow me to tell you a story of how God's Word worked for me one desperate night. A few years ago, while I was attending a grueling and intense week of training for work, I was able to avoid a night-trip to the emergency room by playing Scripture on my laptop.

The previous week, I suffered several wounds on my body from a dog attack, resulting in multiple scratches and bites that caused systemic inflammation. My whole body was swollen and puffy. I was also under a great deal of stress to perform and learn because this was a "make it or break it" sales training. Being out of town, I was not able to eat as healthily as I normally do. Plus, I was sleep deprived from multiple late night training sessions.

On top of everything else, I received a call from someone that was supposed to love me who proceeded to tell me how stupid I was—and it was over a matter that didn't warrant such a response. This person was stressed to the max and decided to unload all of their frustration on me.

Furthermore, I was away from a house where all of my stuff was stored, and it was going to be under permanent lock and key before I could return. This developed after I flew out of state to my week of sales training. I had no idea what was going to happen to my belongings.

While all the other coworkers phoned home to receive loving emotional support from their families for the challenges we were facing, I was confronted with some demeaning, unwarranted verbiage—so I began to crash. I had not been to the emergency room with symptoms of Grave's disease in years, but I recognized my body's warning signs. The disease had returned with a vengeance.

While the group waited for me to come role-play that evening, which was required, I laid in bed trying not to faint. When I tried to get up, I noticed my legs were swelling—as they were simultaneously turning blue. I was so weak and nauseated I couldn't imagine getting in an ambulance. With my bounding pulse racing away, I was too sick to do anything but turn on my laptop.

As I laid there, listening to the Book of Psalms, I meditated on the Scriptures. Finally, my body began to calm down. Eventually, I was able to fall asleep. The next morning, I woke up to a much better mental and physical state. Ultimately, I finished the full seven days of training. It was still one of the most challenging, stressful weeks of my life.

From that experience, I learned the power of listening to Scripture. It is restorative, healing and calming. Sleep can often be a by-product of you listening to Scripture, as opposed to reading the text. When playing Scripture on a handheld device, try to keep the room as dark as possible. For best results, have the temperature cool. Dim the lighting on the screen. Maybe even use earplugs for drowning out disruptive noise.

NEW ASSOCIATIONS WITH SLEEP AND SHEEP

One of the names of God in the Bible is Jehovah Rohi—your Shepherd. In the Scriptures the Lord often refers to you as a lamb—for various reasons. It is no coincidence that our God chose David, a young shepherd boy, to be the King of Israel. Ultimately, Jesus, a descendant of King David, refers to Himself as the sacrificial Lamb—as well as, the Good Shepherd. This means your Creator and Savior relates to you as the lamb you are, while He also comes to you from the perspective of being the Shepherd you need.

During one of my trips to Israel, I visited the "little town of Bethlehem" and toured the fields "where shepherds lay." I loved hearing the actual, modern-day shepherds teach about their relationship with their individual flock of sheep.

Shepherds have always been viewed as one of the lowliest class of people in Bible times. They still are today. But isn't it interesting that Jesus—the Creator of the universe—came to visit the shepherds and the animals first? It's such a paradox; He calls Himself the "Bread of Life," and He was born in a town named Bethlehem, which means house of bread. At birth, He was placed in a manger—the feeding trough for animals. Through the greatest display of humility ever witnessed on the earth, Jesus is telling us, He is our sustenance. Yet, He is the King of all kings and worthy of nothing less than the most splendid palace in the world.

"And she gave birth to her firstborn son; and she wrapped Him in cloths, and laid Him in a manger, because there was no room for them in the inn"
(Luke 2:7).

"Now after Jesus was born in Bethlehem of Judea in the days of Herod the king, magi from the east arrived in Jerusalem . . ."
(Matthew 2:1).

The Bible refers to Jesus as "the Door" to the Kingdom of God. That word picture—worth a thousand words—spoke volumes to the people of that day. It still may speak to you today, but not as clearly, because shepherds are not a part of our daily culture.

At night, after shepherds find a suitable cave, they herd their sheep into the cave and then the shepherd performs an amazing act of love. He lays down across the entrance of the cave, actually becoming—the door—so he can protect his flock from potential predators. This is what Jesus does for you as you sleep. He becomes the Door. If you are His lamb, rest knowing He protects you from harm. But He is also teaching you that He is the Door to Heaven.

So Jesus said to them again, "Truly, truly, I say to you, I am the door of the sheep"
(John 10:7).

"I am the door; if anyone enters through Me, he will be saved,
and will go in and out and find pasture"
(John 10:9).

Each sheep is so precious to the shepherd, he will leave the entire flock to go after that one lamb that is missing. Because a wandering sheep endangers the whole flock, leaving is not be taken lightly. When the lost lamb is found—mostly young sheep tend to wander off—the front legs are broken. Until the legs are healed, the shepherd carries the lamb on his shoulders throughout the day, strengthening the relationship between the lamb and the shepherd.

This teaches the lamb not to wander from the flock again. Your Heavenly Shepherd goes after you like you are His lamb. During your brokenness, He carries you like a lamb and becomes your Lord. Brokenness is the process by which you learn to make Him Lord of your life. Stay close to Him. As you commune with Him, sleep will come.

"All of us like sheep have gone astray,
each of us has turned to his own way; But the LORD
has caused the iniquity of us all to fall on Him"
(Isaiah 53:6).

Shepherds can have different flocks intermingling in the field—with all the sheep grazing next to each other. Then, as individual shepherds start to simultaneously call their own flock, despite the chaos, the sheep will distinguish their own shepherd's voice. It never fails, as dumb as sheep are, each one recognizes its own shepherd's voice and goes straight to its master.

How do they know their shepherd's voice? It's a fascinating phenomenon to consider. All I know is this is how God designed them to behave. This is why, when a shepherd dies, the entire flock has to be killed. The sheep cannot be managed without their shepherd. They only respond to their shepherd's voice.

> *"My sheep hear My voice, and I know them,*
> *and they follow Me"*
> (John 10:27).

David knew all about shepherds and how they tend to their sheep, because he grew up shepherding before he became the King of Israel. It's also why David wrote most of the Book of Psalms. As a lonely shepherd he communed with God. He learned about the ways of God through shepherding his own little flock, and he never forgot these truths once he became King and reigned over Israel.

THE SHEPHERD WHO NEVER SLEEPS SO HIS LAMBS CAN

> *"It is vain for you to rise up early, to retire late,*
> *to eat the bread of painful labors; For He gives*
> *to His beloved even in his sleep"*
> (Psalms 127:2)

Joseph Prince, a prominent, spiritual leader from Singapore, referring to the writings of King David in the Psalms, admonishes you to let go and let God work on all the entanglements of your life—while you sleep. He, who neither slumbers nor sleeps (Psalm 121:3–4), works the night shift for you, while you sleep. Let Jehovah Rohi—your Shepherd, work out the kinks in your life. Allow Him to go before you, throughout the night, to see that you have the guidance and provision you need.

I actually learned another profound truth from Joseph Prince. He tells us that our Promised Land is not a physical territory, as it was in the Old Testament. But our Promised Land, as New Testament believers, is rest. Our Lord is leading us to a place of rest—a state of rest, as a lifestyle.

Prince further reminds us of the story of the Israelites wandering in the wilderness. During this period, God demonstrated that He was the "Bread of Life" in a beautiful manner. He provided manna for His children, as they traveled through the desert from Egypt to the Promised Land. Manna was a form of food much like sweet bread. During the night, the Lord showered the ground with this Heavenly food. It was His perfect provision offered to them each morning. Each new day, they had exactly what they needed—no more and no less.

Because manna was good for that day only, the manna would spoil, if they tried to save it or eat it the next day. This arrangement, by God's design, kept the people dependent on Him for their daily bread. After a while, the Israelites got tired of their manna and began to complain. The manna continued to fall each day, but with the murmuring, it lost its sweetness.

Don't ever murmur against God's daily supply. Your life will lose its sweetness, and part of that is precious sleep. You can sleep soundly throughout the night, knowing your Heavenly Father is providing for you. God's desire is for you to recognize His loving provision, while you sleep, and awaken with an attitude of gratitude. He never slumbers, as He works the night shift. So, you don't have to do anything, but *be diligent to enter His rest*" (Hebrews 4:11). He provides for you during the night and *"supplies all of your needs according to His riches in glory"* (Philippians 4:19).

How do you labor to enter His rest?

There's a delightful story that illustrates this concept about a child at play. While playing outside with her friends, a little girl's necklace gets tangled. She runs into the house and gives the necklace to her mother.

"Mother," the little girl asks without hesitation, "Please untangle my necklace, while I go back out and play." Then, she dashes off again, so as not to miss a moment of fun.

Later that evening, the child's mother hands her the un-tangled necklace. Having completely forgotten about the necklace, the little girl sweetly kisses her mother, as only a child can do and very simply says, "Thank you, Mother." Once again, she is able to proudly display the necklace around her neck.

What is missing in this scenario? There is no begging or pleading for the mother to help her. There is no crying, fret-ting or anxiety over the matter. She innocently believes that her mother is capable and willing to untangle the necklace. She knows and trusts her mother's heart. So, the little girl leaves the tangled necklace, and any care about it with her mother, as she dashes outside to play. She doesn't give it an-other thought, until her mother lays the necklace across the palm of her opened hand—untangled. This is what child-like faith is all about.

There is an inner rest, when you know that all is well. When you are cognizant of a loving Heavenly Father—work-ing through the night to untangle your messy life—you can fall asleep in peace. That is what *"be diligent to enter His rest"* is all about, trusting your Heavenly Father with child-like faith.

Have you heard the old cliché? *I may not know what the fu-ture holds, but I know Who holds the future.* Instead of count-ing sheep to fall asleep, consider the Good Shepherd, your loving Heavenly Father, holding your world in His hands.

Sleep is that sweet part of your day—the benediction—where you surrender the cares of this world and recline into the loving arms of your Shepherd. Instead of counting sheep, realize you are God's little lamb, under His careful watch. He counts the sheep to make sure His little flock is intact, allow-ing you to concentrate on counting your blessings, along with your Zzz's.

I grew up in the Bible Belt with a grandmother who steeped

me in faith—through church, Scripture reading, hymns, and Billy Graham crusades. The following lyrics are from a song we used to sing together:

Count Your Blessings

When upon life's billows you are tempest-tossed
When you are discouraged, thinking all is lost,
Count your many blessings, name them one by one,
And it will surprise you what the Lord has done.
Refrain:
Count your blessings, name them one by one,
Count your blessings, see what God has done!
Count your blessings, name them one by one,
*Count your many blessings, see what God has done.
*[And it will surprise you what the Lord has done.]
Are you ever burdened with a load of care?
Does the cross seem heavy you are called to bear?
Count your many blessings, every doubt will fly,
And you will keep singing as the days go by.
When you look at others with their lands and gold,
Think that Christ has promised you His wealth untold;
Count your many blessings, money cannot buy,
Your reward in heaven, nor your home on high.
So, amid the conflict whether great or small,
Do not be discouraged, God is over all;
Count your many blessings, angels will attend,
Help and comfort give you to your journey's end.

Text: Johnson Oatman, Jr.

Music: Edwin O. Excell

TRUE SHALOM

Whether you are wide-awake, or sleep is settling in, pray over your night. Ask the Lord to come to you in your sleep, protect your sleep, and give you His rest; so you can enjoy dreams of encouragement, course correction, guidance and His nighttime Shalom. In Hebrew, Shalom means, completely whole, with nothing missing and nothing lacking—which includes sleep.

Michael Youssef, *Leading the Way Ministries,* expounds on this idea by talking about the seven aspects of Shalom:

1. Complete well-being

2. Good health

3. Safety

4. Prosperity

5. Favor

6. Tranquility

7. Complete; whole

When you have these seven components of Shalom working in your life chances are you'll be sleeping. Since dreams are one of God's ways of opening your mind to new possibilities, get busy sleeping and dream some dreams. You never know what's around the corner, when you enjoy sanctified sleep. Perhaps there is a dream awaiting you that will take you on a new adventure—just like the adventure Amanda enjoyed.

SCRIPTURES FOR THE SHEEP OF HIS FLOCK

"Sleep" in the Bible

Psalms 4:8
In peace I will both lie down and sleep, For You alone, O LORD, make me to dwell in safety.

Psalms 121:4
Behold, He who keeps Israel will neither slumber nor sleep.

Psalms 127:2

It is vain for you to rise up early, to retire late, to eat the bread of painful labors; For He gives to His beloved even in his sleep.

Proverbs 3:24

When you lie down, you will not be afraid; when you lie down, your sleep will be sweet.

Proverbs 6:22

When you walk about, they will guide you; when you sleep, they will watch over you; and when you awake, they will talk to you (the Lord's principles for living).

Proverbs 19:23

The fear of the LORD leads to life, So that one may sleep satisfied, untouched by evil.

Ecclesiastes 5:12

The sleep of the working man is pleasant, whether he eats little or much; but the full stomach of the rich man does not allow him to sleep.

"Dream" in the Bible

Joel 2:28

It will come about after this That I will pour out My Spirit on all mankind; And your sons and daughters will prophesy, Your old men will dream dreams, Your young men will see visions.

Acts 2:17

'AND IT SHALL BE IN THE LAST DAYS,' God says, 'THAT I WILL POUR FORTH OF MY SPIRIT ON ALL MANKIND; AND YOUR SONS AND YOUR DAUGHTERS SHALL PROPHESY, AND YOUR YOUNG MEN SHALL SEE VISIONS, AND YOUR OLD MEN SHALL DREAM DREAMS;

A SONG FOR SLEEP

Rest

Rest, the Lord is near
Refuse to fear, enjoy His love.
Trust, His mighty power
Fills every hour, of all your days.
Chorus:
There is no need
For needless worry
With such a Savior
You have no cause to ever
Doubt, His perfect Word
Still reassures, in any trial.
Rest, the Lord is there
Lift up your prayer
For He is strong.
Trust, He'll bring release
And perfect peace, will calm your mind.
(Chorus)
Call Him
If you grow frightened
Call Him
With loving care
He'll lift the burden and you'll
Rest, the Lord is near
Refuse to fear, enjoy His love
Trust, His might power
Fills every hour, of all your days
Rest, the Lord is near
Refuse to fear, enjoy His love

Lyrics and Music by Phill McHugh and Greg Nelson
Copyright 1985 River Oaks Music
Co./New Wings Music (a div. of Lorenz
Creative Services Corp.)/ Greg Nelson

SLEEP Q-TIPS:

- The Scripture references in this chapter can be found on this website: http://bible.knowing-jesus.com/Luke/9/32/ type/nasb. Any verse related to sleep; slumber, and dreams can be found on this site, along with the verse concept as it applies to the content and context of the full Scripture reading.

- Listening to Scripture calms your emotions.

- Reading Scripture calms your mind, changing your thoughts.

- Go to www.Penzu.com if you want to download a free dream journal. This site informs you that many of our inventions today were conceptualized first in a dream, i.e., Einstein's dreams led to the creation of his special theory of relativity.

E: THE N.U.R.S.E. APPROACH TO RESTORATIVE SLEEP:

Exercising for Better Sleep

Emotional Fitness Training

Exercises for Breathing Techniques that Promote Sleep

Exercising Joy as the Fruit of Being Rested and Energized

Educating Others to Live Energized and Externally Focused as a Servant

EXERCISING FOR BETTER SLEEP

Not everyone wants to exercise. Some people don't like to sweat. They panic if they even glisten, but others love to work up a big, dripping sweat. Maybe you love exercise and can't wait to hit the gym. Perhaps this is an area of strength in your life, but some people need at least a nudge to get moving.

One of the benefits of incorporating the appropriate amount of exercise into your life is better sleep. According to the National Sleep Foundation, the findings of a recent national study concluded that there is a correlation between physical activity and the overall quality of sleep. It seems that 150 minutes of moderate to vigorous activity per week is the ticket to better sleep.

A nationally representative sample of 2600 men and women, between the ages of 18-to-85, participated in this sleep study about the value of exercise. Here are the findings:

- Sleep quality improved by 65%.
- Participants felt less sleepy during the day by 35%–40%.
- The likelihood of night leg cramps decreased by 68%.
- Difficulty concentrating when tired decreased by 45%.

Basically, they concluded, physical activity helps you feel more alert and less sleepy during the day—with better concentration. This is most likely due to the overall improvement in sleep quality (https://sleepfoundation.org/sleep-news/study-physical-activity-impacts-overall-quality-sleep/page/0/).

If you classify yourself as a sedentary woman, consider this. With just 30 minutes of exercise three times a week, the research shows that you are more likely to sleep an hour longer and wake up less frequently throughout the night (http://www.mindbodygreen.com/0-18647/the-best-time-of-day-to-work-out-if-you-want-to-get-good-sleep.html).

The best time of the day to exercise is up to you. Some people say not to exercise too close to bedtime, suggesting you should have your exercise out of the way an hour before you go to bed. But the benefits are so great, if you find you can exercise, crash into bed, and still sleep like a baby—do what works for you. Perhaps you are able to do a spin class, shower, and jump right into bed with no problem falling asleep. However, if you are like most people, you'll get revved up and be awake for hours. The key is to find what works best for you and go for it.

There are some wonderful phone apps available to help you fall asleep. I am not for or against these apps, but personally I really try to keep my mind free from electronic devices, as I power down for the night. However, the screens on these apps are designed in such a fashion that they do not affect the natural occurrence of melatonin. *Yoga for Insomnia* is one such app. It demonstrates gentle stretches and poses that help the insomniac reach a state of somnolence. For a list of other apps visit:

www.healthline.com/health/healthy-sleep/top-insomnia-iphone-android-apps#.

I cannot emphasize to you enough the connection between sleep and exercise. Sleep is vital to living a healthy, optimal lifestyle. Right behind it is exercise; they work in tandem. Sleep restores and repairs, while exercise acts as a pump for the lymphatic system. Lymph nodes are scattered throughout the body as key warriors in the fight against potential infections—toxicities that you encounter on a regular basis. If you are healthy and your lymphatic system performs correctly, you will never know about these infections, because your immune system effectively wards them off.

Unlike the circulatory system, where the heart pumps blood throughout the body, the lymph system has no pump for the lymphatic system. Your body's lymph system needs your exercise as the pump for the system. Otherwise, the lymph system stays static—just like a swamp. A clogged lymph condition results in signs and symptoms of inflammation and infection, which lead to all sorts of problems—including chronic fatigue, arthritis, headaches, eczema, skin conditions, water retention, cellulite, obesity, allergies, and the list goes on.

As you age, you no longer breathe from your abdomen like children. You breathe more shallowly from your chest, which does not allow for needed oxygenation of the blood. The ability to force circulation of lymph fluid throughout the body is solely a function of deep breathing. Exercise causes you to breathe deeply, and it is extremely important that you breathe this way for optimal health.

EXERCISES FOR BREATHING TECHNIQUES THAT PROMOTE SLEEP

Andrew Weil, MD, author of *Spontaneous Healing*, writes about an amazing breathing technique that works wonders in helping you fall asleep. I highly recommend this for insomniacs. Here are the doctor's breathing instructions for this exercise:

- Exhale completely through your mouth, while making a whooshing sound.
- Close your mouth and inhale quietly through your nose to a mental count of four.
- Hold your breath for a count of seven.
- Exhale completely through your mouth, making a whooshing sound to a count of eight.
- This is one breath. Inhale again, repeating the cycle three times, totaling four breathing cycles.

Note: Your inhalations should be quiet, while you breathe through your nose. Exhalations should be audible through the mouth, with the tip of your tongue positioned against the ridge of the tissue just behind your upper teeth. This should be done throughout the entire exercise. Exhalations should be twice as long as inhalations. This exercise acts as a natural tranquilizer. So, practice this breathing technique as often as you need to and for as long as you like. Dr. Weil has more therapeutic breathing exercises to try, so visit his website for more techniques: http://www.drweil.com/drw/u/ART00521/three-breathing-exercises.html.

If you do this right, the most obvious benefit of exercise will be looking better and maintaining your youth. Stretching keeps you flexible and more limber, while staying at a good size gives you a more youthful appearance. A toned, fit body is sexy. Who doesn't feel more confident when they are in shape?

As a confident person, you are more engaging and successful on the job, and especially more sexually attractive to your partner. But exercise can be overdone and lead to joint problems. So, it is important to find what works best for you. Listen to your body. It will alert you, if you are overdoing it, or you need to rest. Be wise enough to know what your body is telling you and comply with its message.

You should heed the warnings your body sends through pain and inflammation, which is often a direct cause of insomnia. When choosing a form of exercise as a beginner, or a regular participant returning to activity, be gentle with yourself and find your groove. As you begin to know your abilities and limitations, you can push yourself accordingly.

When you are rested from a good night's sleep, exercising regularly and consuming good nutrition, you are more likely to inhale plenty of oxygen and keep it flowing through your body. Consequently, you are more apt to sport a joyful essence, exuding more positive energy. You even smile a great deal more. Keep in mind, out of 53 total facial muscles; it only takes thirteen muscles to smile but 47 to frown. Different sources vary slightly on this but this is the general consensus.

EMOTIONAL FITNESS TRAINING

You've probably heard of the expression wearing your

heart on your sleeve. This phrase has a negative connotation, implying you don't have control of your emotions. Wearing your heart on your sleeve—and wearing unattractive facial expressions—both signal that something is missing in your life. Don't allow that missing component to be sleep, which is a by-product of unresolved toxic emotions.

In her book, *Twelve Easy Emotional Fitness Exercises*, Katherine Gordy Levine, M.S.S. LCSW, reveals new research findings, supporting evidence that you can give your emotions a "workout" through emotional fitness training. You can actually identify a specific emotion and through emotional fitness training, you can develop emotional muscles—helping you to overcome and conquer negative emotions that cause you to behave badly.

Look more closely at Levine's groundbreaking book. It is masterful at helping you manage any toxic emotions that might be keeping you up at night, thereby adversely affecting your ability to fall asleep or stay asleep throughout the night.

In another book with a similar concept, *Cleansing Made Simple*, Cheryl Townsley conveys, when it comes to your physical health, two of the most debilitating emotions you can experience, are fear and anger. Here is Cheryl's list of emotions, correlating with specific bodily organs and a few of their resulting maladies:

- Anger—settles in the liver
- Fear—asthma, respiratory problems and upper chest tightness
- Bitterness—gall bladder
- Guilt—shoulder problems
- Control or hatred—colon
- Loneliness—aches

- Suppression—allergies
- Hostility or unforgiveness—arthritis
- Inadequate finances—lower back problems
- Resentment—candida
- Despair—chronic fatigue
- Nervousness—coughs
- Need for protection—weight
- Stress—headaches
- Grief—lupus
- Inflexibility—multiple sclerosis
- Irritation—skin problems
- Insecurity—stomach problems

Other resources may offer a more in-depth or exhaustive list, but this one shows a basic compilation of the specific bodily organs, where emotions settle, and the potential consequences of living with these unresolved issues. You have to be diligent in your emotional fitness training—in order to promote emotional health—so that you are free from emotional toxins. (Refer to this matter in the R section, where we explored more of what might be keeping you up at night.)

Fitness training, whether emotional or physical, boosts your spirits and lifts your mood. The benefits are endless for you and for those who cross your path.

EXERCISING JOY AS THE FRUIT OF BEING RESTED AND ENERGIZED

Hopefully, the physical fitness bug will bite you and infect you with a true love for exercise. Try the following creative ideas, as a jump-start to your physical activity. See if you don't sleep better at night and demonstrate a more joyful disposition:

1. Walk your dog without your ear plugs, while paying attention to him or her.

2. Run two steps and skip on the third for as long as you can (Fun to try on the beach.)

3. Jump on a trampoline, large or small. (Rebounding is fun.)

4. Ride a bike through the woods.

5. Visit another country on a stationary bike while reading a book or watching a movie.

6. Tap-dance; it works wonders for the legs.

7. Try yoga to build an unbelievable body and clear your mind.

8. Sign up with a pilates instructor for a long, lean, beautiful body.

9. Like a ballerina, use a bar for a long, lean, and toned body, with exceptional definition.

10. Hand weights. Keep them in the car with your walking shoes. The world becomes your gym.

11. Walk the treadmill, while watching TV or reading a book. Kill two birds with one stone. Catch up on favorite programs, while you are doing something healthy.

12. Swim like a kid. It's great for the joints!

13. Stretch to keep young and flexible—especially while in bed, before rising for the day.

14. Planks are great for core and strength building.

15. Knee squats increase testosterone.

16. Lunges are an excellent way to firm and tighten the tops of your legs.

17. Walk four miles in one hour, five days a week, with your stomach tucked in. You will lose 20 pounds by year's end—with no other changes to your lifestyle!

18. Buy a Hula-Hoop and get rid of your waist, kid-style.

19. Learn to belly dance.

20. Zumba!

21. Go on a hike. Maybe join a hiking group.

22. Roller skate or ice skate.

23. Stand up and sit up straight, holding your stomach in throughout the day. As you practice good posture, it makes you look younger, and it is very healthy for your internal organs. It also helps fight shallow breathing.

24. Shake it off!

25. Ballroom dance.

26. Use arm bands or weights by the ocean, in a park, or while watching a chick flick.

27. Paddle boat across the lake.

28. Jump rope!

29. Water slide.

30. Climb a wall—inside or outside.

31. Take the stairs at every opportunity.

32. Park as far away as possible from the entrance of your destination and walk more every day.

33. Dance like no one is watching—forget that it's cliché, it's fun!

34. Power walk in Sketchers.

35. Snow ski.

36. Water ski.

37. Shoot a basketball.

38. Go horseback riding. Women in the north that ride, have tight inner thighs. While riding tightens the thighs, the freezing cold temperatures freeze that fat between the legs. Some horse farms need people to ride their horses and will actually pay people to come and saddle up.

And the list goes on . . .

Eric Liddell: "I believe God made me for a purpose, but He also made me fast. And when I run I feel His pleasure," *Chariots of Fire.*

Some of my favorite ways to exercise are:

- Jumping on the trampoline
- Dancing
- Power walking on the beach
- Practicing water ballet in the pool or water aerobics
- Walking my dogs
- Snow skiing, but I seldom get to do it.

These activities help me feel God's pleasure. They also allow me to offer my body as a living sacrifice—whole and perfect—in an act of worship to God.

One final note—According to Gayle Green—author of Insomniacs, and the blog, Sleep Starved, "Sleep is the fuel of life. It's nourishing; it's restorative. And when you are robbed of it, you are really deprived of a basic kind of sustenance." You've seen this quote before, if you read the Nutrition section, but I believe repetition is the mother of retention.

Make your own "smorgasbord" list of activities that cause you to feel God's pleasure, when you exercise. Get the soles of your feet moving and avoid being sleep starved with some real foot stomping "sole food." You will sleep so much better.

What is "sole food?" It's feeding your soul by moving the soles of your feet; exercising so that oxygen is pumped right to the cell, giving energizing sustenance. This is important because God has a call on your life, and you need to be physically prepared and well rested for the assignment.

Your Creator does not want you to walk around half dead. He wants you fully alive, living a life that brings Him joy. Did He not say to offer your body as a living, holy sacrifice? This means He wants you to take care of your earthly suit—He calls it the *Temple of the Holy Spirit*. It does not glorify Him, or benefit you and the people you serve, to walk around fat, bloated, inflamed, full of pain, diseased and tired.

"Therefore I urge you, brethren, by the mercies of God, to present your bodies a living and holy sacrifice, acceptable to God, which is your spiritual service of worship"
(Romans 12:1).

When your parents or important guests come for a visit, you spiff up the place, and remove anything controversial; you really deep clean. A mani-pedi and a hair trim most likely make the list of self-improvements, because you want to look your best. Perhaps you prepare a favorite recipe they really appreciate. You probably get your car detailed, if you own one, because you want to present yourself in the best possible light—while making them feel special during their visit.

The Creator of the world wants to reside inside you much like a hand in a glove. He deserves the same effort, if not more, than an important visitor to your home.

His Holy Spirit desires to indwell your heart, mind and

soul; leading and guiding you to live the life He designed for you to live. Through His coexistence and internal promptings for wise living, you will eat right and exercise a little every day. Do whatever it takes to get restorative sleep. Make your body—the temple of His Holy Spirit—a beautiful, clean dwelling place for your Creator, so that He can enjoy His rule and reign in your life. Together, as you abide by His Kingdom principles, you'll be empowered to live an abundant, joyful, satisfying life, full of sweet sleep.

EDUCATING OTHERS TO LIVE ENERGIZED AND EXTERNALLY FOCUSED AS A SERVANT

When you are rested and participate in energizing exercise on a regular basis, along with the right nutritional plan—you can focus on others and not just on your own sleep-deprived misery. Helping others is a form of worship. Setting a good example, while helping others, empowers you to enlist more servants in a world that tends to feel lousy because of poor life-style choices.

Taking care of yourself and modeling a healthy life-style within a sick world that desperately needs your help, is like the infamous mother on a crashing plane that places the oxygen mask over her mouth, before assisting her child. It's vital that she have oxygen, so she can be strong and available for those depending on her. Take care of yourself, so you can focus on others.

An even higher calling than role modeling healthy life-style choices is actually taking the time to teach others. Rather than just handing someone a fish because they are hungry, I believe in setting them free by teaching them how to fish. Teaching someone how to achieve what you have already achieved, as a role model, is the highest form of love. I am not a proponent of dependency, whether it is a sleeping pill or any other form of dependency. I'm for empowering you to make wise, rewarding, and liberating choices, so that you can drive and manage your own destiny.

There is one exception to this issue of dependency. I am 100% in favor of being completely surrendered to the in-dwelling power of the Holy Spirit. Much like the hand in glove reference that I alluded to earlier. Being controlled and dependent on Him is the ultimate way to live.

I invite you to welcome God into your life. Let Him live in your heart and empower you to live optimally, so that you can become outwardly focused. (See the Exchanged Life Prayer: Appendix A.) Make your body, which is His dwelling place, the best it can be. He will get the glory, and you will reap the benefits. By following this principle, you can be a little Mother Teresa in your own tiny corner of the world. You can go to bed at night with a smile on your face, knowing that you made the world a better place in some small way, because you remembered to reach out to others rather than only think of yourself.

SLEEP Q-TIPS:

- No matter what activity you choose, double up and do two things at once to save time and improve your quality of sleep. Do sit-ups while you catch up on cable news or any other exercises you choose, such as walking on the tread-mill or riding a stationary bike.

- Play some TobyMac music—you can't help but move when you hear it.

- Go to any one of several websites, enter your weight, the length of time you exercised, along with the chosen activity, to calculate the total number of calories you burned.

- Because you have your own unique gifts to offer the world, take care of yourself by getting enough sleep in tandem with exercising, so you can be available to help others through role modeling and educating.

CONCLUSION

Congratulations, you've survived your first adventure with me as your nurse coach, based on The N.U.R.S.E. Approach to Restorative Sleep. We started the journey together, with me addressing you in a very militant manner, but all in good fun. Initially, concerning the matter of sleep, I was very firm, because choosing to live a well-rested life, in this day and age, takes intentionality and fortitude.

We live in a complex world that seems to be unraveling at the seams, but going without sleep helps no one—you must sleep. Consider me to be your mama bear taking that mean old "insomnia beast" down.

Sometimes, when life gets too serious, it's helpful to approach your challenges in a fun—not so grim manner—thus, the purpose of our fictitious character, Amanda, from the movie, *Holiday*. As she remodeled her life, due to debilitating insomnia, my own sleep-deprived life paralleled with her script. I decided to use her storyline to convey some very sobering scenarios regarding sleep loss, as well as, share with you ways to tackle the underlying causes of what may be keeping you up at night.

Ultimately, Amanda made an exchange that changed her life. I offered you an exchange in this book that not only cures insomnia but also gives you a chance to change your entire life profoundly and eternally.

As we went along, I eased up a bit, hoping you'd feel my coaching style shift from militant to that of a loving parent, tucking you into bed for a wonderful night's sleep on the "magic carpet" of dreams. Obviously, this is the softer side of my inner mama bear.

My hope is that you'll grab some Zzz's, so you can be energized to live your life optimally and present your best-rested self to a world that desperately needs your finger print on the global landscape.

Oops! Duty calls, I have someone calling me at this very moment.

"Nurse, Nurse, I'm Worse! Can you help me sleep?"

I want to hear wonderful reports from all of you, as you incorporate the N.U.R.S.E. Approach to Restorative Sleep, into your way of living and sleeping.

Find out what's keeping you up at night and kick insomnia out the door, forever, through:

Nutrition

Uncluttering

Remodeling

Spirituality, and

Exercise

Good night and sweet dreams!

Contact me at: NurseNurseImWorse!@gmail.com

APPENDIX: A

The Exchanged Life Prayer

Lord Jesus,
I know I am a sinner.
No matter how good of a person I think I am,
It does not meet Your standard of perfection and holiness.
Please forgive me of my sins.
I believe You shed Your blood for me as a ransome,
Because You love me more than I can possibly comprehend.
You lavishly paid for my sins and rescued me from poverty,
fear, disease, and insomnia.
You have given me eternal life, a future and a hope.
Please take over my life and allow
Your Spirit to dwell within me.

I trust and follow You as my Lord and Savior.
Guide my life and help me do Your will.
Impart to me Your abundant life.
Please send me friends that know You and will help me grow
In my walk with You, so I can enjoy sweet sleep
and fulfill my destiny.
Help me take care of myself, so I can be available
to help others along the way.

In Your name, the name above all names, I ask this,
Amen.

APPENDIX: B AMANDA'S CARE PLAN

ASSESSMENT	PLAN	IMPLEMENTATION	EVALUATION
Nursing Diagnosis: *Insomnia* related to anxiety (as evidenced by difficulty falling and remaining asleep, fatigue, and irritability).	• Examine Amanda's coffee intake and sugar intake. • Do a nutritional evaluation.	Have Amanda complete the Adrenal Fatigue Quiz as referred to on pg. 30. Use the N.U.R.S.E. Approach to Restorative Sleep to help examine the following categories::	Sleep [0004] as evidenced by: • Sleeps through the night consistently • Feels rejuvenated after sleep
Subjective: "I can't cry and I can't sleep...I hear work jingles in my head all night... All I do is work, work, work..." "My life is out of balance...my boyfriend is gone because of it..." "Can someone help me?"	• Examine her exposure to hand held devices. • Set up a routine to quieten her mind starting at sundown so she can power down.	**Nutrition:** Her problem is not secondary nutrition but primary nutrition. **Un-clutter:** • Her bedroom - It is a sanctuary for sleep and intimacy. • Her mind - through routine and mental exercises..	• No dependence on sleep aids • Able to dream and recall the dreams, as well as journal dreams • Clear supple skin
Objective: Height: 172.72 cm (5'8") Weight: 54.43 kg (120 lbs.) Temperature: 37.00C (98.6 F) Pulse: 78 BPM Respirations: 16/minute Blood pressure: 120/74 mm Hg	• Drill down and identify problems with the five pillars of rest.	• Her heart - by *remodeling her life, through the Exchanged Life. ***Remodel:** the five pillars of rest, by removing toxic people from her life and getting away from the rat-race to rejuvenate with a house-swap.	• Bright eyes absent of bags and puffiness • Smiling with a peaceful disposition. • Energized
Diagnostic Data: CBC within normal limits, Normal chest x-ray Bags under eyes with dark circles, acne, dehydrated skin		***Spiritually:** incorporate Scriptures into her daily routine and set apart sleep for dreaming, not rehearsing work jingles. REM sleep is vital. *Exercises:* for 1) the physical, 2) the emotional and 3) breathing —to energize. Experience the Exchanged Life, Appendix A.	